The Daily Telegraph

MIGRAINE

D1461448

The Daily Telegraph

MIGRAINE

VALERIE SOUTH

ROBINSON
London

Constable & Robinson Ltd
3 The Lanchesters
162 Fulham Palace Road
London W6 9ER
www.constablerobinson.com

First published in Canada by Key Porter Books Limited, 2000

First published in the UK by Robinson,
an imprint of Constable & Robinson Ltd, 2002

A copy of the British Library Cataloguing in Publication Data
is available from the British Library.

ISBN 1-84119-475-1

Printed and bound in the EU

10 9 8 7 6 5 4 3 2 1

*To my husband, Bob, whose unwavering support
helped make this book possible,
and
for my sons, Mitchell, Cameron and Thomas.*

*In memory of the first migraine sufferer
I knew – my mother, Mabel.*

Contents

Foreword

Migraine is amongst the most baffling of all illnesses. Its classic specific symptoms of a crushing unilateral headache have, after all, been recognized for the best part of 2,000 years, ever since their first description by the Roman physician Aretaeus in the second century AD. Numerous doctors and scientists have written learned treatises about it while the range of possible treatments – both preventive and for the acute attack – is enormous. Yet, the question 'what is really going on here?' remains unanswered.

There is, in short, no unifying theory of migraine, so much so that it appears it must involve processes that lie beyond the ability of medical science to explain. There has been, it is true, and as Valerie South lucidly explains, a fundamental shift in recent years away from the vascular theory that invokes the restriction and subsequent dilation of the blood vessels in the skull as the final common pathway of a migrainous attack. Rather, the radically different hypothesis currently being proposed is that the problem lies in the brain stem connecting the brain to the spinal cord, from which, it is claimed, nervous impulses pass backwards along the sensory nerves from the face to produce migrainous type symptoms. This theory would seem to be supported by sophisticated brain scanning studies providing some rationale for the effectiveness of the latest, and most expensive, of anti-migraine drugs, the triptans – through their effect on the neurotransmitter chemical serotonin. It cannot be said, however, that this new theory has significantly deepened our understanding of the condition.

It is necessary to recognize medicine's profound ignorance about these matters if we are to appreciate the virtues of a more practical approach to the condition. There are, as pointed out, a wide range of possible treatments for migraine, most of which have been found to influence the severity or frequency of major attacks quite by chance. We may know no more about why they should work than the underlying processes of migraine itself, but there is every reason for those afflicted to learn about them, 'just in case' they might prove to be effective.

I have received several letters from readers of my *Telegraph* medical columns over the years pointing out how their migraines have 'disappeared' after, for example, having been prescribed the betablocker drugs for angina or calcium antagonists for raised blood pressure, or indeed after starting Prozac or amitryptilene for depression. Others have variously described discovering for themselves how their attacks can be aborted by a hot sweet drink (or even just a glass of hot water), by ice cubes, by tying a tight bandage around the head or by plucking a few leaves from the feverfew plant and eating them in a sandwich to conceal their bitter taste.

Valerie South's *Migraine* includes a most comprehensive summary of this range of treatments whose value can so readily be overlooked in the current enthusiasm for the triptan drugs. Triptans have proved of enormous benefit to many patients, but it is worth remembering that they are only one of a variety of treatment options. All of those afflicted with migraine, it is to be hoped, will learn something useful about their baffling illness from the experience of Valerie South and the several other contributors to this volume.

Dr James Le Fanu
London, 2002

Preface

I have migraine. Quite possibly you or someone you know is also affected by migraine. Migraine affects at least 10 per cent of the UK population, yet around 60 per cent of migraine sufferers have never consulted their doctor. One study asked doctors why they thought their migraine patients came to see them. Most believed that their patients came primarily to obtain pain relief. But when the patients responded to the same question, most said that the main reason they came to the doctor was to seek help in understanding their pain.

Migraine is a misunderstood disorder that often goes untreated or is improperly treated by patients and their health-care providers. There is even a common belief that migraine is an imagined disorder and that sufferers bring the symptoms on themselves out of a desire for attention. This belief can force those with migraine to suffer in silence.

This book is intended to be helpful to all migraine sufferers and those close to them. It offers in-depth information in understandable terms on the medical nature of migraine and answers a need for up-to-date, relevant information on the status and treatment of migraine.

The information provided in this book is intended to be general and should not be used as a tool for self-diagnosis or as a substitute for medical treatment. To ensure their own safety and good health, readers must always consult a doctor before embarking on any treatment or therapy, including those described in this book and elsewhere.

Readers should be advised that any treatment, therapy, or opinion described in this book should not be interpreted as medical advice or recommendation. Any mention of a commercial product, medication, therapy or treatment of any kind does not represent an endorsement from any of the parties involved in this book. Drugs are identified by generic (chemical) name, and when brand names are given they are examples only. Note that many drugs are sold under different names in different countries, and that new drugs are constantly appearing.

It is my pleasure to present this book to migraine sufferers in the hope that it will bring strength and understanding to all concerned. The assistance provided in the chapters that follow can be hard to find in a society that often tells the victims of migraine that their pain is 'all in their heads'.

Valerie South

1
Understanding Migraine

Migraine is a medical disorder that is prevalent around the world. It affects 8–14 per cent of people in developed countries and is similarly or somewhat less prevalent wherever else its scope has been examined. Most surveys suggest that migraine affects 10–15 per cent of the population. In the UK alone, if you consider a working population of about 38 million adults, about 3.8–5.7 million people have migraine. However, this is only an estimate, as it is difficult to assess the exact incidence and prevalence of the condition. A study published in the medical journal *Neurology* in 1999 found that migraine may affect up to 33 per cent of women and 13 per cent of men at some time during their lives.

Headache is one of the most common medical complaints, and yet migraine remains a poorly understood malady. It is troublesome that, despite current knowledge, sufferers often do not seek help. This may be because they think that nothing can be done for migraine, or perhaps feel as if their condition will not be taken seriously by the doctor. Furthermore, about one-third of migraineurs and only one-quarter of doctors correctly recognize the headache as migraine, with obvious consequences on management. Yet, migraine is not, by any means, a new phenomenon.

A historical perspective

Headache is as old as the human species itself. Writings dating back to the beginning of recorded history indisputably describe the symptoms of migraine. Aretaeus of Cappadocia, a medical writer in the second century, is believed to be the first person to have recognized a one-sided headache disorder involving stomach upset and visual disturbances. Shortly thereafter, Galen, a contemporary of Aretaeus, and a court physician to Marcus Aurelius in Rome, termed these headaches 'hemicrania', meaning 'one-half of the head', after the type of pain typically experienced by many migraine sufferers. Later, the Old English term 'megrim' emerged. Finally, the word 'migraine', adopted from the French, evolved.

For centuries, doctors, scientists and researchers have tried to unravel the mystery of migraine, and have developed a variety of treatments in the process. For instance, drilling holes in the skulls of people with migraine to release the evil demons believed to be responsible for the headache was a common and often deadly practice as early as 7,000 BC. (Bone regrowth at the edges of the wounds in more than 50 per cent of the skulls found suggests that some of the victims lived for a time after the procedure.) The *Papyrus Ebers*, dating from about the sixteenth century BC, describes the Egyptian crocodile treatment for migraine. The treatment involved strapping a clay crocodile to the top of the sufferer's head with a piece of linen bearing the names of the gods. An offering of grain to the gods was laid in the crocodile's mouth. The treatment may have actually brought a small measure of relief to the sufferer, as the weight of the crocodile and the pressure exerted by the linen straps would have compressed inflamed blood vessels and nerves in the scalp.

The medical treatment of migraine began in 400 BC, when the Greek physician Hippocrates, the so-called 'father of medicine', described attacks of visual disturbances, head pain and vomiting typical of migraine. He noted that these headaches could be brought on by exercise or sexual intercourse, and could be partially relieved by vomiting. (Many migraine sufferers today agree with these observations.)

During the thirteenth century, severe headaches were treated with poultices of opium laid upon the skin. The absorption of the opium through the skin was enhanced by the addition of vinegar to the poultice.

Throughout the years many artists with migraine have depicted both the visual disturbances that accompany many attacks and their personal images of the pain experienced. One such artist was Hildegard of Bingen, a nun who painted what she believed to be divinely inspired visions in 1180. Her paintings, entitled *Visions of the Fall of the Angels*, capture the visual warning signs, or the aura, that accompanied her migraine attacks.

It was not until the seventeenth century that knowledge of medicine and the human body let physicians speculate more accurately about the causes of disease. One of the most important physicians in the history of neurology was Thomas Willis, who published *Cerebri Anatome* in 1664. In that work, he documented elements such as diet and atmospheric changes that he knew could trigger migraine in susceptible individuals. Willis's writings point to alterations in blood flow within the brain associated with migraine. Later termed the 'vascular theory of migraine', Willis's theory was not challenged until recent times, but is now considered too simple to explain the exact cause of migraine. Out of Willis's discovery of the role of blood vessels came Erasmus Darwin's (grandfather of Charles Darwin) centrifuge treatment for migraine. Held by their hands, Erasmus's patients were swung in a circle in an effort to force blood away from the swollen migrainous blood vessels in the head. Had any of Erasmus's patients been around about 200 years later, they would have surely preferred William Gowers's prescription – smoking marijuana.

William Gowers and Edward Liveing challenged Thomas Willis's vascular theory of migraine with their belief in the neurogenic theory of migraine. Liveing published the first major work devoted to migraine, titled *On Megrim, Sick-headache and Some Allied Disorders: A Contribution to the Pathology of Nervestorms*, in 1873. Liveing and Gowers believed that migraine originated from electrical 'nerve storms' within the brain and that the disorder was closely related to epilepsy.

Recently, it has come to light that a previously overlooked doctoral thesis by Elizabeth Garrett Anderson, written three years before Liveing and Gowers and entitled 'Sur la Migraine', may have been one of the first significant papers demonstrating profound understanding of migraine coupled with sound practical advice for sufferers. First translated into English in 1966 by Dr Maria Wilkinson, this paper helped set the pattern for treatment at the City of London Migraine Clinic over the last thirty years. In the clinic there is emphasis on the need for regular meals, a regular schedule and the treatment of attacks with rest, plenty of hot tea and simple analgesics combined with anti-emetics.

It is surprising that, despite its long history, migraine was not the subject of scientific laboratory study until the 1930s. Using volunteer migraine patients, an American doctor, Harold G. Wolff, conducted experiments that supported the vascular theory that the pain of migraine is caused by the overdistention of blood vessels in the head. There is no question that all migraine sufferers have Dr Wolff to thank for propelling the study and treatment of migraine forward, but Dr Wolff may also be responsible for giving migraine sufferers a bad reputation. Until the twentieth century, migraine had always been perceived as a *bona fide* medical disorder. Today migraine sufferers are often accused of making up their symptoms to gain attention, or of not being able to handle what non-enlightened people believe to be simply minor discomfort.

Wolff observed that the patients he saw in his lab had certain personality traits in common. He coined the term 'migraine personality', describing these patients as 'rigid, perfectionistic, controlled and orderly, overly conscientious, fearful of making mistakes, while they seek approval from their environment'. Wolff's publicizing of this opinionated belief has done an immense injustice to migraine sufferers. Dr Wolff's observations were more likely a mere coincidence, and studies conducted since then fail to prove or disprove his statements consistently. The migraine sufferers involved in Dr Wolff's work perhaps more notably shared a willingness to have surgery done under local anaesthetic so that Dr Wolff could expose their scalp arteries, dilate the vessels with clamps and attach threads to their artery walls in the name of medical research.

There is no such thing as a migraine personality. We've all encountered people who seem to be the personification of stress – mug of coffee in one hand, cigarette in the other, screaming into a telephone while a taxi waits outside – yet who have never had, and will never have, a migraine attack. On the other end of the scale sit many migraine sufferers who are the most laid-back, gentle people one could ever imagine. No one 'type' or group is singularly susceptible to migraine; it affects people of all ages, races, cultures, personality types, occupations and income levels.

The prevalence and impact of migraine

Chances are everyone knows someone with migraine, be it a friend, family member or a colleague. Famous migraine sufferers in history include Sigmund Freud, Frédéric Chopin and Thomas Jefferson. Lewis Carroll, author of *Alice's Adventures in Wonderland*, was a migraine sufferer, and many believe that his migraine aura provided inspiration for the content of the book, as well as for many of the illustrations done under his supervision. Other famous sufferers include Michael Aspel, the late Princess of Wales and sports figures Roger Black and Steffi Graf. But how much sympathy do the almost one in five people who suffer from migraine receive when they fall ill with it? Not much, according to most people with migraine. Perhaps migraine tends to be overlooked because it is so common and is not deadly (although it can ruin life). Perhaps because it is not contagious, people without migraine don't fear or respect it as much as they do other disorders. The fact is, migraine can be a very serious medical disorder that significantly affects the person with the condition, and his or her immediate family, friends, employers and colleagues.

The mental exercise in the box on p.7 may help you get a glimpse of the world of the migraine sufferer. Imagine that in addition you are likely to encounter someone who clearly

Imagine that . . .

If you do not have migraine but are trying to understand the effect on those who do, reading this book is a good start. It may also be helpful for you to try the following mental exercise to put you somewhere near being in the shoes of a person with migraine.

Imagine the impact that repeated episodes of a particular illness would have on you and those around you. First, with each episode you feel ghastly. It may not always be possible, despite dramatic physical illness, to lie in bed when the routine responsibilities of life must be attended to. You may be forced to drag yourself out of bed, to attend to the needs of others as well as your own. After all, your symptoms occur so often that your loved ones can't always be there to pamper you. Perhaps you may be able to call in sick to work, but what if you have called in sick often enough for your employer to be concerned about your attendance? What if this is your second or third bout of illness this month? Or what if you have an important deadline to meet, and your boss and colleagues doubt the validity of your illness? You may be able to take medication, but you often find the side effects of the pills make you unable to do your job or drive a car. You find it hard enough just to think and speak, without adding a medication haze to your day. And what about those theatre tickets you have for tonight? You'll have to be the one to drop out again, as well as absorb the non-refundable cost of the tickets.

thinks, 'Oh, you're probably just faking,' or says, 'Take a couple of painkillers and get down to business,' when you return to the office.

Migraine strikes at work, at home and at play. A study of 845 people with migraine showed that they report a lower quality of life than those with other health problems such as angina, diabetes mellitus or a previous heart attack. Another study showed that 78 per cent of people with migraine report that they cannot carry out their normal activities as well during their attacks. The mean number of attacks experienced was twenty per year. Eleven per cent of the people in the study reported one or more headaches per week. The data also show that, of the migraine attacks experienced, 17 per cent were associated with cancellation of a family or social activity and 11 per cent were associated with an absence from work.

The last thing a person with migraine will do when an attack hits is call in to work sick. The first things to go are family activities like cooking, cleaning, grocery shopping and spending time with partners or children. Next, social events are cancelled. It's not surprising that 75 per cent of those with migraine modify their behaviour because of the effects migraine has on their interpersonal relationships and the limitations it imposes on their lifestyle. But it is not until a significant portion of their lives is already affected that a typical sufferer will pick up the phone to call in to work sick.

When we look at the economic impact of migraine on the workplace, we must think of the additional personal costs as well (the taxi to get home when one is too sick to drive, the bill for the take-away food for the family when one is too nauseated to cook, the cost of medications and other treatments, etc.). Nevertheless, migraine costs the economy a loss in productivity *in the workplace alone* amounting to an estimated £612 million in the UK each year. This estimate is based on conservative figures. A mere 'take two tablets and call me in the morning' headache could certainly not have this type of impact on individuals or the economy!

What is migraine?

Almost everyone experiences a headache now and then. Usually it is a result of stress, fatigue or worry; for some it is a result of an overindulgence in alcohol (a hangover). These headaches are a result of the normal make-up of the human body. Other headaches are actually a symptom of another problem such as those caused by infections or tumours.

Migraine differs from both types of headaches as it is an actual medical disorder itself.

Migraine's symptoms range from moderate to severe, and one study showed that 31 per cent of the migraine attacks experienced forced the sufferers to stop daily activities or to go to bed. Migraine involves head pain for some, dizziness for others. Some will have nausea; some will be bothered most by an inability to form words or to concentrate. The variety of symptoms that can be caused by migraine has made it poorly understood and underdiagnosed. The complexity of the neurobiochemical processes that underlie migraine, and in turn cause the many different symptoms, fascinates researchers. Migraine will show up in one person as a certain collection of symptoms; a different collection of symptoms will present themselves in the next. Nevertheless, the cause is the same.

No one knows the root cause of migraine, although more has been learned about what goes on in the body of a migraine sufferer in the last ten or fifteen years than ever before. As well, migraine has been defined and described, and clinical criteria developed by the International Headache Society (IHS) now aid in the identification and diagnosis of migraine and other types of headache disorders. While researchers are working towards finding all of the answers, we do have a strong base of knowledge to begin with.

Migraine tends to run in families, which suggests it may be an inherited disorder. One survey found that 66 per cent of people with migraine report that a close blood relative suffers from similar headaches and in 53 per cent of these cases the relative is their mother. Others who can't readily identify a relative with migraine may remember a grandmother or great-aunt who complained of 'bilious attacks' or 'sick headaches'. These were probably migrainous. My paternal grandfather practically lived on aspirin (acetylsali-cylic acid) for pain, plus a mixture of baking soda and water for the nausea associated with his frequent sick headaches. (This same grandfather was once thought a lazy boy trying to avoid his farm chores as he often had to lie down in a field on his way home from school until his headache eased.) In light of migraine's familial tendency, extensive genetic research is being carried out worldwide. From earlier studies we also know that in the case of twins, approximately half of the susceptibility could be attributed to genetics, and half to environmental factors. In the mid-1990s there was an extremely important discovery of gene mutations on chro-mosome 19 and 1. These mutations seem to be a factor in 70 per cent of cases of a rare form of migraine known as familial hemiplegic migraine (the remaining 30 per cent remains unaccounted for). Geneticists continue to study chromosome 19.

What causes the symptoms of migraine?

For decades, the pain of migraine has been thought to have a vascular origin (to originate in the blood vessels). Until quite recently, many migraine sufferers were told that the single cause of their migraines was a constriction (narrowing) of the blood vessels in the head, which caused warning signs, or an 'aura', such as visual disturbances for some, followed by a painful dilation (widening) of the blood vessels, which caused the headache. That blood vessels play a significant role in migraine is still generally accepted in the medical community, but the events in the body and the resultant symptoms associated with a migraine attack are now proven to be too complex to be associated solely with constriction and dilation of blood vessels. Although it is difficult to explain what is known about migraine today without using medical terminology, it is important to have some understanding of the medical complexity of migraine.

Some doctors tell patients with migraine that they have a 'raw central nervous system' that is prone to migraine and is very sensitive to external triggers. However you think of it, the central nervous system of a person who gets migraine is different from that of a non-sufferer. Migraine sufferers have a biochemically based medical problem in their nervous system that makes them very prone to a specific set of symptoms known as a 'migraine attack'. The degree of proneness to an attack can vary, resulting in infrequent attacks in some, and frequent attacks in others. The attacks may be set off in response to what are known as 'migraine triggers'. These triggers may be external (such as the chemical content of certain foods) or internal (such as the release of particular hormones). We will discuss triggers later.

Migraine is a brain disorder, and all of its symptoms – including the pain, nausea, vomiting, aura symptoms, etc. – come from within the nervous system. Although blood vessels are certainly involved, results of tests using sophisticated technology such as magnetic resonance imaging (MRI) and positron emission tomography (PET) scans have led scientists to de-emphasize the prominence of their role. Yet absolute agreement in the scientific community tends to end there. While some researchers look to areas of the brain such as the brain stem for a 'migraine generator', others study the role of chemical messengers such as serotonin (pronounced sarah-toe-nin) and dopamine (see Chapter 2 for warning symptoms which may suggest migraine's association with dopamine deficiency). Another group of researchers point to pain-producing substances such as substance P, calcitonin-gene-related peptide

(CGRP) and neurokinin A. A system involving the nerve that your dentist has likely had occasion to 'freeze' in order to perform dental work – the trigeminal nerve – is another suspect in migraine.

Those studying the 'migraine generator' include a group in Essen, Germany, led by Dr Hans Diener. These scientists have used PET scanners to study changes in blood flow within the brain during and after an attack, as well as between attacks. Increased blood flow was shown in two areas of the brain. Subsequent treatment with a medication that mimics certain actions of serotonin relieved the pain and symptoms of the migraine attack and returned blood flow to normal in one of these areas (the cortical region) but *did not* return the blood flow to normal *within the brain stem*. Some researchers believe this means that the activity within the brain stem during the attack may not be the result of the headache, but may be somehow more critically involved. This finding may explain why this group of serotonin-mimicking medications (the triptans – see Chapter 9 for more on these) can relieve symptoms. (The brain stem is very rich in serotonin.) But despite initial relief through manipulation of serotonin using triptan medications, many people find that the attack later returns because the medication hasn't turned the 'migraine generator' off.

Serotonin (known chemically as '5-hydroxytryptamine', or '5-HT') influences many bodily functions such as mood, sexual arousal and appetite. It has a wide spectrum of effects on the nervous system, gastrointestinal system, respiratory system and cardiovascular system. It is made by the body from an amino acid called 'L-tryptophan', a substance found naturally in foods such as milk and turkey. It may be a raised serotonin level which makes a warm drink of milk before bed feel relaxing, or a big holiday turkey dinner feel comforting. Natural tryptophan levels in human breast milk may bring added comfort to infants.

Although the exact role serotonin plays in a migraine attack is still debated by researchers, depletion of serotonin in the brain is believed to be linked to migraine. Circulating levels of serotonin rise at the beginning of a migraine attack as the serotonin is moved from its proper location into the bloodstream. Levels then fall dramatically when the attack is in progress as the serotonin is removed from the bloodstream and excreted from the body in the urine. There are believed to be at least seven main types of serotonin receptors throughout the body. These receptors are found in the central nervous system, as well as in the gut (the two areas of the body most affected during a migraine attack).

Medications can control certain symptoms by altering the effects of serotonin on particular receptors or subtypes of receptors. For instance, since depression is an illness associated with low levels of serotonin, researchers discovered that by using medications that work on both serotonin and other receptors (via a complex mechanism not yet fully understood), we can reduce the depressive symptoms. In migraine, the same action with the same medication has the effect of preventing migraine attacks! Same medication, same action, but when the medication is used for a different disorder (sometimes at a different dose) you get different effects. That is why some migraine sufferers benefit from taking an antidepressant at low doses – it helps with migraine; it's *not* being prescribed because the doctor secretly believes the patient is depressed. It was also recently discovered that, by stimulating certain subtypes of the $5\text{-}HT_1$ receptor site ($5\text{-}HT_{1B}$ and $5\text{-}HT_{1D}$) with medication that mimics certain actions of serotonin, it may be possible to abort the symptoms of a migraine attack in progress. So you see that, although it is complex and not fully understood, the role of serotonin in migraine is a very important one. Conclusive evidence of the impact of serotonin on migraine comes from the observation that, if a migraine sufferer is injected with the drug reserpine, which causes a depletion of serotonin from the body's stores, a migraine attack results. This artificially induced headache can then be stopped by injecting pure serotonin back into the bloodstream (although doing this causes serious vomiting, making it an unacceptable treatment for migraine).

Some researchers spend a great deal of time looking at the *trigeminovascular system* – the one linked to the dentist's favorite nerve to freeze, which includes the membrane covering the brain and spinal cord. This system communicates messages from the migraine generator to blood vessels and other structures in the head, and pain is caused by the inflammatory response. This inflammation is caused by the other chemicals of interest in migraine – substance P, CGRP and neurokinin A. These chemicals have nasty effects, similar to those of a bee sting, on the nerve endings surrounding the blood vessels. The area becomes inflamed, swollen and tender – and the pain of migraine results via stimulation of the pain-sensitive nerve endings.

Finally, suspicions about disruptions in blood flow to the brain are not entirely cast aside by the new way of thinking. Blood flow has been demonstrated to decrease in the back areas of the brain during a migraine attack and this reduced activity spreads gradually forward across the brain during the beginning phases of the headache and/or during the aura. The blood flow across the brain is reduced for a few hours before returning to pre-headache levels. Similar changes in electrical activity are seen in the area of the brain controlling visual responses – perhaps explaining visual auras. Other auras such as numbness or tingling, difficulties with speech, etc., may be due to similar disruptions in other areas of the brain.

What exactly sets off this long and complicated cascade of events is sometimes difficult to pinpoint. We know that the predisposition to attacks comes from having the disorder itself – very likely owing to the person's genetic make-up. We also know that the cascade *can* be set in motion by 'triggers' that tend to be very individual, but that often work in combination to somehow weaken the defences sufficiently to allow the abnormal process that culminates in a migraine attack to begin. The trouble is that the triggers are not always obvious and are often hard to avoid – such as menstrual periods or other hormonal factors. More will be said about triggers later.

But there remains one unanswered question – *why?* Although we have genetic evidence for predisposition, and information about what is happening during an attack, we have yet to nail down undisputed causes or cures. The importance of continuing the quest for knowledge about migraine cannot be overstated.

Dr R. Gordon Robinson, a neurologist and migraine expert from Canada, explains a migraine as follows:

Migraine is now accepted as a biological disorder of the brain similar to other recurrent painful disorders of other organs such as angina and heart disease. It is believed that individuals go though life with a degree of headache proneness, often inherited, that is dictated by an area deep within the brain rich in a neurotransmitter called serotonin. Changes within this area may be precipitated by trigger factors occurring either from the outside (bright lights, weather changes, etc.)

or within the individual (hormonal fluctuations, sleep disruptions, etc.). These may set in motion a complex neurochemical phenomenon which may produce changes within other areas of the brain to create aura, often in the form of visual phenomena. The same system acting via nerves to the head and neck is responsible for producing the typical pounding/one-sided headache of migraine. The actual pain of the headache appears to be produced through a combination of swollen blood vessels and inflammation in tissues within the head and neck as well as the lining of the brain. These changes are also dependent upon serotonin activity in the region. Hence, migraine is a many-faceted disorder produced by the brain itself acting upon other areas within it as well as other areas of the body, including the stomach.

2
Diagnosing Migraine

Despite its prevalence and impact, migraine is one of the most under-recognized, misdiagnosed, and mistreated medical problems today. Statistics show that 46 per cent of migraine sufferers who go to a physician about their headaches will receive an improper diagnosis. This is hardly surprising, given that the average undergraduate medical student receives only minimal formal education about migraine. Another reason may be the common misperception that migraine is not a legitimate illness. This attitude toward migraine may force sufferers of frequent headaches into seclusion in the belief that they must learn to live with their attacks. Many sufferers resort to medicating themselves, and may actually further damage their health as a result. Worse yet, migraine sufferers may fear that their doctor will minimize their complaint if they seek medical help. Of those who had been to see a doctor, one study showed that 45 per cent were no longer doing so. Only 36 per cent ever returned for ongoing care. Those who stopped seeing a doctor often cited negative experiences as a main reason. They thought their doctors were not interested in or knowledgeable about headaches and didn't view headaches as a valid medical complaint. Others in the study said they gave up going to the doctor because of problems with the medications that were prescribed. A survey released in 1999 showed that, in the US, patients tried nearly five treatments on average before being offered an effective one. Most of the sufferers who turned away from the medical profession resorted to self-medication, which resulted in poor pain relief.

These facts underscore the importance of migraine education. Migraine sufferers must have the ability and opportunity to become informed, empowered participants in their own care, in partnership with knowledgeable, caring physicians. And the first step in gaining control over migraine lies in obtaining the proper diagnosis.

The symptoms of migraine

Many people think 'migraine' is just a fancy term for a bad headache. In fact, migraine is a *bona fide* medical disorder, and its symptoms are far more wide-reaching than head pain.

In 1988, the International Headache Society (IHS) published a document that was formulated by the best migraine specialists from around the world. The document grew out of a need to standardize the definition of various types of headaches. Without such a tool, one doctor might see a headache patient and diagnose 'tension-type headache' or might prefer to use other terms for the same thing, such as 'muscle-contraction headache' or 'stress headache', while a second doctor would diagnose migraine in the same patient. A standard set of definitions was also needed so that data from migraine research projects could be compared. Without such a tool, one researcher would be collecting information on apples and another on oranges. Outside of the research lab, this 96-page document is a little unwieldy. Nevertheless, when diagnosing headache, the doctors we see today apply a practical interpretation of the very valuable information compiled by the IHS.

Migraine without aura

Of the seven main types of migraine, the two most common are migraine with aura and migraine without aura (an aura being a warning sign). The IHS's description of migraine without aura (formerly called 'common migraine'), published in their journal *Cephalalgia* (Volume 8, Supplement 7, 1988), reads:

> Idiopathic [cause unknown], recurring headache disorder manifesting in attacks lasting four to seventy-two hours. Typical characteristics of headache are unilateral [one-sided] location, pulsating quality, moderate severity, aggravation by routine physical activity and association with nausea, vomiting and/or photophobia [light sensitivity] and phonophobia [sound sensitivity].

In other words, migraine without aura is a recurring headache disorder that is not caused by another underlying problem such as a tumour. The pain of migraine tends to throb or pulsate, and usually (but not always) occurs on one side of the head. The pain is often made worse by physical movement, and is usually moderate in intensity. Other symptoms can include nausea, vomiting and sensitivity to sound and/or light.

*Adapted IHS definition of migraine without aura**

A. At least five attacks have occurred, fulfilling items B–D, below.

B. The headache lasts four to 72 hours if not treated, or if the treatment used doesn't work.

C. The headache has at least two of the following characteristics:

1. one-sided pain

2. pain pulsating with the heartbeat

3. pain of moderate or severe intensity

4. pain made worse by physical movement such as climbing stairs

D. During headache, at least one of the following other symptoms is also present:

1. nausea and/or vomiting

2. sensitivity to light and sound

E. There is no evidence of another underlying disease.

It is important to point out that it is possible to diagnose migraine without aura even though *not every potential symptom is present*. For example, someone suffering from migraine without aura need have only two of the symptoms listed under C and only one of the symptoms listed under D. The variability of symptoms may explain why so many people find it hard to understand migraine, and ask how two people with the same disorder can have different symptoms.

Migraine with aura

Migraine with aura (formerly called 'classic migraine') is the second most common form of migraine. Approximately 20

* Adapted from *Cephalalgia*, Volume 8, Supplement 7, 1988.

per cent of migraine sufferers will experience a neurological warning sign, or aura, before the symptoms of their attack occur. It may not happen with each attack and the warning sign may vary from attack to attack. For many, the aura will come as a visual hallucination such as zigzag lines across the visual field. For others, it will be a true blind spot before the eyes. The visual problems originate in the brain, not in the eye. Other auras originating from the brain may include a numb, tingling feeling in the tongue and fingertips (known medically as 'digitolingual paraesthesia').

*Adapted IHS definition of migraine with aura**
A. At least two attacks have occurred, fulfilling item B.
B. The attack has at least three of the following characteristics:
   1. One or more temporary aura symptoms are present that actually stem from an area within the brain.
   2. At least one aura symptom develops gradually over more than four minutes, or two or more symptoms occur right after each other.
   3. No aura lasts longer than 60 minutes. If more than one aura symptom is present, this length of time increases proportionally.
   4. Headache follows aura within sixty minutes (it may also begin before or at the same time as the aura).
C. There is no evidence of another underlying disease.

In plainer English, migraine with aura is diagnosed in a person who has had at least two attacks with a warning sign. The warning sign must have at least three of the four following characteristics:

* Adapted from *Cephalalgia*, Volume 8, Supplement 7, 1988.

1. The aura must be one that causes symptoms generated from within the brain, such as visual hallucination. These symptoms must be temporary.
2. The symptoms 'blossom', developing gradually over a period of more than four minutes. A second symptom may develop immediately after the first, causing a slower 'bloom'.
3. Individual symptoms of the aura last no longer than sixty minutes after they first appear.
4. The actual headache and other symptoms of migraine follow the warning within sixty minutes. The headache may also begin before or at the same time as the aura.

As well, migraine with aura is diagnosed only when there is no other disease present which would cause these symptoms. Once again, we can see that, since only *three* of the four characteristics under item B are necessary to diagnose migraine with aura, two people with the same diagnosis may experience it in different ways.

The aftermath of migraine

Although post-attack symptoms are not recognized by the IHS, most migraine sufferers agree that, even after an attack has passed, subtle symptoms remain for an additional day or so. Referred to by many as the 'hangover' (although it has nothing to do with alcohol consumption), the period immediately following a migraine attack can leave the sufferer feeling spent. Often there is a need to rest and extra sleep is reported to help some. Other symptoms of the aftermath may include a depressed mood, difficulty concentrating, tenderness of the head, neck-ache or neck stiffness, reduced physical abilities

Other symptoms that are not auras

The aura should not be confused with another set of symptoms that can precede *any* form of migraine attack, known as 'premonitory symptoms'. Premonitory symptoms may be related to the brain chemicals dopamine and serotonin and usually occur in the 24 hours before the attack begins. Commonly these symptoms can include:

- hyperactivity – sometimes manifesting in an unusual desire to make the house spotlessly clean, or unusual talkativeness (known as 'the Chatty Cathy syndrome')
- exaggerated feelings of well-being or excitement
- hunger and/or a craving for a particular food (commonly sweets or chocolate)
- thirst
- increased sexual desire
- depression, irritability or other unexplained change in mood
- difficulty concentrating
- excessive yawning
- drowsiness.

The premonitory symptoms can be so subtle that they are not recognized by the sufferer until brought to his or her attention by family members or close friends.

and clumsy arms and legs. The good news is, once all the symptoms of migraine and its aftermath pass, many report that just feeling 'normal' again is a pleasant relief.

Other types of migraine

The other five types of migraine and the subtypes of migraine with aura are less common but can be as, if not more, distressing. Since they are so rare, discussion of the details of these less common types will not be lengthy. However, a listing and brief description of the associated symptoms may be helpful. It is also important to know that it is believed that the same mechanism that gives a person so-called

IHS types of migraine

1. Migraine without aura
2. Migraine with aura
    2.1 Migraine with typical aura
    2.2 Migraine with prolonged aura
    2.3 Familial hemiplegic migraine
    2.4 Basilar migraine
    2.5 Migraine aura without headache
    2.6 Migraine with acute onset of aura
3. Ophthalmoplegic migraine
4. Retinal migraine
5. Childhood periodic syndromes that may be precursors to or associated with migraine
    5.1 Benign paroxysmal vertigo of childhood
    5.2 Alternating hemiplegia of childhood
6. Complications of migraine
    6.1 Status migrainosus
    6.2 Migrainous infarction
7. Migraine disorder not fulfilling above criteria

From *Cephalalgia*, Volume 8, Supplement 7, 1988.

typical migraine also causes the more uncommon forms of migraine. Therefore, many of the treatments of uncommon migraine will be the same as for the more common forms of migraine.

Below we briefly examine the symptoms of the other types of migraine.

Migraine with prolonged aura (formerly 'complicated migraine', 'hemiplegic migraine')

This occurs when one or more aura symptoms last longer than one hour but less than a week, and investigative scans are normal. Aura symptoms can include visual hallucinations, numbness or tingling in hands and weakness in limbs.

Familial hemiplegic migraine

This occurs when the aura symptoms include a one-sided weakness (almost paralysis) and at least one immediate relative has identical attacks. The one-sided weakness may be prolonged.

Basilar migraine (formerly 'basilar artery migraine', 'Bickerstaff's migraine', 'syncopal migraine')

The aura of this migraine includes two or more of these symptoms:

- visual symptoms in both the inside visual field (toward the nose) and the outside visual field (toward the temple)
- slurred speech
- dizziness (vertigo)
- ringing in the ears (tinnitus)
- decreased hearing
- double vision
- unsteadiness on feet
- numbness and tingling in limbs on both sides
- severe weakness/paralysis of limbs on both sides of body
- decreased level of awareness of surroundings.

Migraine aura without headache (formerly 'migraine equivalents', 'acephalgic migraine')

This type of migraine involves a typical aura, but *no headache*. It is common from time to time for any sufferer of migraine with aura to have the aura with no subsequent headache. It can become more common in these sufferers as they age, and in fact the headache may stop coming altogether in the older sufferer. If, however, migraine-aura symptoms without the headache begin to occur for the first time in people over the age of fifty, special laboratory investigations may be done by the doctor to rule out other possible causes such as transient ischaemic attacks (TIAs), or 'mini-strokes'.

Migraine with acute onset of aura

In this type of migraine, the aura fully develops in less than five minutes. A typical migraine headache follows.

Ophthalmoplegic migraine

This very rare type of migraine involves repeated headaches with a paralysis of one or more cranial nerves that control eye movement and the size of the pupil. Symptoms may include double vision.

Retinal migraine

In this type of migraine, the sufferer's aura involves a temporary blind spot or total blindness in *one eye only*, lasting less than sixty minutes. Retinal migraine usually involves a headache before, during or within one hour after the blindness ends.

Childhood periodic syndromes (formerly 'migraine equivalents')

Childhood periodic syndromes include 'benign paroxysmal vertigo of childhood', in which an otherwise healthy child experiences many short attacks of loss of balance, anxiety and sometimes shaking of the eyes back and forth or vomiting. Another syndrome is called 'alternating hemiplegia of childhood' and involves attacks of extreme one-sided weakness/ paralysis, alternating from side to side in infants less than eighteen months of age. It also involves other abnormal posturing, body movement and abnormal brain function. This disorder may be more closely related to epilepsy.

Complications of migraine

Two main types of complications occur frequently enough to be defined. The first is known as 'status migrainosus' – a headache that lasts more than 72 hours without a break in the pain for longer than four waking hours. This type of headache is usually associated with prolonged use of certain symptomatic medications (usually narcotic painkillers). Sufferers in the throes of status migrainosus often require drug treatment aimed at breaking the attack. Treatment is usually given in a hospital's emergency department, and if dehydration is present, fluids may be given intravenously.

The other main type of complication is frightening but rare, and is known as 'migrainous infarction'. This type of migraine is associated with one or more aura symptoms that continue for seven days or more. The symptoms are caused by a migraine-related stroke. However, research shows that stroke is a *very rare* complication of migraine.

Other migrainous disorders

Finally, headaches that are believed to be a form of migraine but do not fit the so-called textbook definition may be recognized as having a migrainous origin under the title 'migraine disorder not fulfilling above criteria'. This provision allows doctors to form an opinion about whether the patient's collection of symptoms that do not exactly match a set of IHS-defined criteria for migraine is indeed migraine-related. Other migrainous disorders can produce symptoms that are not fully typical of the more common types of migraine. For instance, some people may experience bouts of feeling detached, vaguely nauseated or unsteady on their feet, and actually be suffering from a form of migraine. Migraine can cause troubling dizziness for some, or difficulty with concentration for others. These symptoms and others may or may not be accompanied by headache, and are thought to be caused by the same neurobiological alterations present in typical migraine. Indeed, migraine can have many different faces. The existence of this category underscores the importance of seeing a physician for proper diagnosis, and avoiding self-diagnosis based on the information given in this book, or elsewhere.

Helping your doctor with the diagnosis

> English, which can express the thoughts of Hamlet and the tragedy of Lear, has no words for the shiver or the headache. The merest schoolgirl when she falls in love has Shakespeare or Keats to speak her mind for her, but let a sufferer try to describe a pain in his head to a doctor and at once language runs dry.
>
> – *Virginia Woolf, 'On Being Ill'*

Explaining what migraine is by listing symptoms or

describing the scientific reasons why migraine occurs is very different from explaining to someone what migraine feels like. Although one person's experience of a particular set of migraine symptoms will differ from another person's, people with migraine agree that their problem demands to be taken seriously. Some migraine sufferers are able to press on, with difficulty, during their attacks, while some will be forced into bed, with the curtains drawn and the telephone unplugged. Migraine can be treated, but the first step toward conquering migraine involves obtaining a proper diagnosis and enlisting the help of the medical profession in the process.

Migraine is diagnosed solely on the basis of what the patient tells the doctor. There is no blood test for migraine. Sophisticated scans and tests will not 'show' migraine (although they are sometimes done as part of the diagnosis to rule out the existence of other neurological problems). Migraine is evaluated on what is known as a 'clinical diagnosis'. The doctor takes the information on symptoms provided by the patient and applies specific diagnostic criteria. As we mentioned, if there is some overlap with the symptoms defined in the IHS criteria, the doctor's diagnosis may well be migraine, even though the symptoms aren't 'textbook perfect'. Most of the symptoms of migraine are subjective; that is, since no one can tell from the outside what another person is feeling inside, the doctor can't measure the pain of migraine or see the warning signs a patient with migraine with aura may feel. For this reason, it is imperative that migraine sufferers be clear, concise and exact when describing their symptoms to their doctor. It is not enough to say, 'I've been having headaches lately.'

People with migraine must help their doctors gather all the necessary information. Many people expect their doctor to draw out their symptoms by asking questions. This type of interrogation works well in police work, but isn't the best approach in medical care. Migraine patients know what their symptoms are and how they are feeling, and they are the best people to describe both. It's a good idea to take a piece of paper and a pen, and jot down *all* the symptoms experienced with the attacks before arriving at the doctor's office. This will help you to recall information, since you are most likely to seek medical attention in between attacks, while you are pain-free. As well, having a list will help you to be confident and clear, since many people find they tend to 'go blank' in the doctor's office. Compounding the problem is the feeling of being rushed when visiting the doctor. The waiting room may be full of people while the doctor zooms from one consulting room to another. Although it is important to be organized in order to make appropriate use of the doctor's time, it is also essential that the doctor take time to listen carefully to the patient. Patients must try not to let the fast pace of the doctor's office get to them; taking a deep breath will help in slowing down. The doctor will listen, and is responsible for taking the time to give the attention so strongly needed for the proper diagnosis and treatment of headache. If a migraine patient does not have the full attention and concern of the doctor, it is up to him or her to find a doctor who will listen, and with whom a trusting relationship is possible.

If you get migraines, helping your doctor with his or her powers of observation is critical. The doctor may be the world's most knowledgeable about migraine, but can't apply that knowledge to you without having as complete a picture as possible. The 19th-century writing of Charcot and Féré (which, coincidentally, deals with the subject of migraine) emphasizes the importance of the physician's ability to observe the patient. The following is an excerpt translated writings originally dated 28 February 1888:

> Let someone say of a doctor that he really knows his
> physiology and anatomy, that he is dynamic – these
> are not the real compliments; but if you say he is an
> observer, a man who knows how to see, this is per-
> haps the greatest compliment one can make.

Communicating the disability associated with migraine

In recent years, it has become clear that it is highly effective
for people to describe to their doctors the disability associated with migraine as a way of 'painting a clearer picture'

Prepping for your appointment

It may be helpful to complete this list of questions and to communicate
your answers to your doctor in order to help with the diagnosis of your
headache type:

1. How frequently do the attacks occur?
2. When did the attacks begin?
3. Where is the pain located?
4. What does the pain feel like (e.g., stabbing, dull, throbbing, pressure, etc.)?
5. What makes the headaches worse?
6. What makes the headaches better?
7. What do the attacks prevent you from doing?
8. What other symptoms are there (e.g., nausea, visual disturbances, sound sensitivity)?
9. How long do the attacks last?
10. Does there appear to be any pattern to them or something that 'triggers' them (e.g., food, weather, fatigue, menstrual cycle)?
11. Do any family members also suffer from similar attacks?
12. What medication (if any) has been taken? How frequently? Did it help?
13. What other therapies or measures have been tried? Did any help?

of what it is like to live with migraine. The impact that migraine and other headache disorders have on one's quality of life has until recently not been well recognized or appreciated.

Useful tools have been developed as an effective aid to better doctor–patient communication regarding disability. Studies have shown that, once equipped with information regarding impact and disability, physicians perceive a migraine patient's needs with more urgency, and assign resources more effectively to address the problem. Patients don't readily volunteer this information, nor do doctors routinely ask for it – hence the need for the development of tools easily accessible via the internet, such as the MIDAS instrument (www.midas-migraine.net) and the Headache Impact Test (www.amIhealthy.com).

Once he or she has considered all the information supplied about the attacks, the doctor will formulate an opinion about the diagnosis. If the symptoms fall outside the range of what would be considered consistent with migraine, and there is even a slight chance that the attacks could be happening as a result of some other malfunction within the body, the doctor may choose to order investigative tests. The laboratory tests described below will not confirm migraine, and are not done routinely. As a matter of fact, the tests will be 'negative', or normal, if the diagnosis is migraine. The tests may, however, rule out the presence of other neurological problems.

The neurological examination

The neurological examination is always done on patients with suspected migraine. This examination is performed in the office and is completely painless and non-invasive. The doctor is able to learn a lot about the brain's functioning through simple techniques that test reflexes, strength, co-ordination, orientation to surroundings and time, certain visual abilities and sense of touch.

Blood tests

There is no blood test available to determine whether or not a person has migraine, but blood tests can sometimes tell if the problem isn't migraine. Other disorders that can cause headaches will cause abnormalities in the blood that can easily be screened for as part of a routine check-up to rule out health problems other than migraine.

X-rays

Plain X-rays have limited value in the diagnosis of head pain. But some structures outside of the brain can be seen with a plain X-ray, such as the sinuses and neck. The doctor may order X-rays to rule out sinus infection, neck injury, arthritis or other such disorders and conditions.

The CAT scan

The CAT scan (computerized axial tomography scan, or CT scan, as it is sometimes known) is probably the most common 'extra' evaluation done to rule out more sinister causes of head pain such as tumour, stroke or bleeding. It is not routinely done to diagnose migraine because, if the diagnosis is truly migraine, the results of the CAT scan will be negative, or normal. This scan is done to detect the presence of potentially life-threatening causes of head pain.

CAT scans are quite sophisticated and somewhat expensive.

They are not available at all hospitals, and there may be a waiting list for those needing one on a non-emergency basis. The patient lies on a narrow table and his or her head is surrounded by a donut-shaped scanner. The procedure is painless, but it may be uncomfortable to lie perfectly still while the image is being taken. For some, contrast dye will be injected into a vein to enhance the picture. Risks involved are minimal, but include exposure to X-ray radiation at only slightly higher levels than in skull X-rays, and the possibility of an allergic reaction if contrast dye is injected (particularly in people with an allergy to shellfish).

The MRI

MRI (magnetic resonance imaging) is the most recently developed type of scanner, and is available in even fewer hospitals than are CAT scanners. It is usually done to find out more about a problem that was noticed on a CAT scan. Since migraine does not show up on CAT scans, MRI is rarely done in cases of migraine. It may be done more often in future as budgets and technology allow, to diagnose non-migrainous problems such as aneurysms (ballooning of the blood vessel). However, MRIs done in the name of research on migraine patients show that they may have more normally occurring small white lesions in the brain than do those without migraine. No one knows the meaning of these lesions as yet. They may mean nothing and be purely coincidental. Research in this area is continuing.

Transcranial Doppler studies

Transcranial Doppler studies use an ultrasonic device (a transducer) to painlessly measure changes in the rate of blood flow through major arteries in the head. They may detect a narrowing of arteries in the head if blockage or spasm is present. These studies were traditionally done for research purposes only, but recently are being done more frequently in patients with migraine. Some clinicians question the value of performing Doppler studies in all migraine patients, and the results of the tests will not prove the presence of migraine. (A clinician is a doctor who works at treating patients, rather than at research or some other medical function.) Nevertheless, Doppler studies are non-invasive, and may pick up certain coexisting problems.

The EEG

EEGs (electroencephalograms) are done as part of the headache check-up only when there is some suspicion about the cause of unusual aura symptoms, or where the doctor has a hunch that seizure activity could be a factor. The EEG is performed in a laboratory; wires are taped to the patient's head, and brain waves are monitored on a screen. It is a painless, non-invasive procedure.

Lumbar puncture

The lumbar puncture, or spinal tap, is done as part of the diagnosis only when severe infection, bleeding or a change in the pressure of the fluid surrounding the brain and spinal cord is a possibility that is being considered. This procedure involves 'tapping' a small amount of fluid from the space around the spinal cord, using a needle. The skin in the area is anaesthetized to reduce the discomfort. Sometimes a small meter is used to measure the pressure of the fluid.

Other tests

From time to time, the doctor may order other tests to rule out coexisting health problems. Patients may be asked to consider undergoing laboratory evaluations when voluntarily participating in migraine research studies. Evaluations may include angiography (X-raying blood vessels after dye has been injected) or PET (positron emission tomography) scans. These tests will, once again, not necessarily show migraine, but will help to pinpoint any other problems that may be present, or to evaluate research.

3
Headaches – Not Migraines?

In addition to the seven types of migraine discussed in Chapter 2, there are several other types of non-life-threatening headache disorders. Although the differences between the rigidly defined types of headache may seem small, or purely academic, they are actually quite important. The treatments used for the different types of headache disorders often vary. In this chapter, we examine forms of headache that are not migraine but may be somehow related to migraine, or may be present in people with migraine.

Tension-type headache

Almost everyone experiences so-called tension headache from time to time. This type of headache is usually mild to moderate, and it isn't usually necessary to see a doctor about it. Often people describe the pain of a tension headache as the feeling of wearing a hat that is too tight, sometimes with a feeling of tension in the shoulders and back of the neck. The pain usually disappears by itself, or with the help of non-prescription pain relievers, rest, relaxation or even a cocktail at the end of a stressful day (by comparison, alcohol will often worsen a migraine). It used to be believed that this type of headache was caused by the contraction (tightening) of the muscles around the head and in the neck as a result of stress. For this reason, this type of headache also used to be called 'stress headache', or 'muscle-contraction headache'. Measurements of muscle contraction in the scalps of people with migraine often reveal a higher level of contraction than in the scalps of those with tension headache, so even the term 'tension headache' is misleading. Many researchers now believe that the mechanisms underlying tension-type headache may be related to migraine. Some believe that tension-type headache sits at one end of a continuum, and migraine at the other.

The International Headache Society has renamed tension headache as 'tension-type headache'. Episodic tension-type headache does not occur regularly and does not usually interfere with plans at work or at home. It is described by the IHS as: 'Recurrent episodes of headache lasting minutes to days. The pain is typically pressing/tightening in quality, of mild or moderate intensity, bilateral in location and does not worsen with routine physical activity. Nausea is absent, but photophobia or phonophobia [sensitivity to light or sound] may be present.'

If these headaches occur more often than 15 days per month (180 days per year), they may be described as 'chronic tension-type headache'. This type of headache is present for at least six months. The headache is usually pressing/tightening in quality, mild or moderate in severity, bilateral and does not worsen with routine physical activity. Nausea, photophobia or phonophobia may occur. This type of headache can be debilitating. Frequently, it evolves as episodic tension-type headaches become more frequent. It can also evolve out of migraine.

Tension-type headache and migraine

There is mounting evidence that when tension-type headache occurs in people with migraine (migraineurs) it may be a 'different beast' than episodic tension-type headache. People with migraine often experience tension-type headaches that are more frequent, longer and more severe than those seen in people who don't also have migraine. Interestingly, the newer 'triptan' agent sumatriptan, custom-made to treat migraine, has been reported to be helpful against tension-type headaches in migraineurs. Sumatriptan also works against chronic tension-type headaches (but not against episodic tension-type headache in non-migraineurs), pointing to a different mechanism for these disorders than for episodic tension-type headache alone.

Other daily headaches

During the past decade or so, researchers and clinicians have realized that the IHS classification failed adequately to outline a very common problem seen in headache clinics worldwide – headaches that occur every day or almost every day.

Other terminology has since been proposed to more effectively describe the different daily headaches. For instance, some people start to experience daily headache without a history of migraine or tension-type headache, and this is termed 'new daily persistent headache'. Perhaps more commonly, daily headache can actually evolve out of migraine:

someone affected by migraine may begin to experience additional daily or almost daily headache with different – often milder – features. First described as 'transformed migraine', this phenomenon is associated with milder (in comparison with migraine head pain) chronic headaches that do not usually interfere with daily activities but make the days less enjoyable. Sufferers usually have less energy for a social life and can become depressed. Sleep disturbances, anxiety and loss of interest in sex are also common.

Migraine on its own has the capacity to turn into chronic daily headache. However, periodic migraine can be transformed into chronic daily headache when prescription or non-prescription pain relievers are taken too frequently. If these medicines are used no more than three days per week, they can be helpful. But if any amount of them is taken on four or more days per week, they will worsen migraine. Often the vicious cycle of overuse of pain relievers begins quite innocently with a couple of tablets taken here and there. But as the low-lying, almost ever-present tension-type headache continues, many people develop a need to take more and more tablets. As tolerance to the medication develops, the amount needed to obtain the same degree of relief quickly escalates. Many people falsely believe that the headaches are not severe enough to see the doctor. They may also falsely believe that any amount of non-prescription medication is safe to take. In actual fact, daily headache is a serious problem and requires medical attention. Other terms used to describe chronic daily headache associated with overuse of medication are 'medication-induced headache', 'rebound headache' and 'analgesic-withdrawal headache'. In this book we will use the term 'medication-induced headache', or MIH. Perhaps it is the growing awareness of this disorder that accounts for the inconsistencies in names. In any case, many doctors and authors recognize the need to standardize the terminology.

The cycle of medication-induced headache

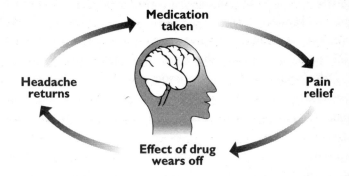

Medication-induced headache occurs when regular doses of pain relievers are taken. The pain relievers actually cause chemical disruption in the brain, which results in a daily, or almost daily, underlying headache. When the pain relievers are taken on four or more days a week over a period of time, the body 'gets used to' this amount of medication, and its level of natural painkilling endorphins shrinks. MIH can happen with even the mildest forms of pain reliever, as well as with the stronger prescription narcotics (a form of MIH can also occur after a sudden withdrawal from caffeine). Since MIH can happen with the smallest amount of medication taken on a regular basis, cutting down to one or two pills every day is not adequate prevention. It is also not good enough to substitute one type of pain reliever for another, or to substitute a non-steroidal anti-inflammatory or migraine-specific medication for the pain reliever. Use of any type of symptomatic (as opposed to 'preventive' or 'pro-phylactic') medication for migraine must be limited to fewer than four days per week. As well, preparations containing the drug ergotamine should be taken only as directed by the prescribing physician. Overuse of ergotamine can cause toxic side effects as well as the rebound effect.

The type of brain sensitivity associated with medication-induced headache occurs only in headache sufferers. Arthritis sufferers who take pain relievers daily do not develop MIH. Neither do sufferers of other types of persistent pain disorders.

Other factors that may be associated with the change from episodic headaches to chronic headaches include stress, traumatic life events, personality factors, high blood pressure and certain medications.

People who suffer from daily or almost daily headaches and who find themselves digging into the pill bottle almost every day can feel isolated and alone. They often avoid reaching out for help for fear that their painkillers will be taken away, although their pills are giving them slight, temporary relief at best. Others fear being called 'drug addicts'. These fears are natural, but headache sufferers who are caught in the vicious cycle of overuse of pain relievers are not addicts. They ended up in the cycle out of a desire to obtain relief from a painful medical problem.

There is hope for sufferers of medication-induced headaches, but much of the healing can and must be done by the sufferer, with some help from the doctor.

The first step in the management of medication-induced headache involves recognizing the problem. The overuse of medication is a subtle and insidious problem, and most people are unaware of the amount of medication they are taking. By keeping a note of how many pain relievers are being consumed, people with MIH will see that they are likely taking medication more than three days per week. Taking pain relievers for three or four consecutive days during a single episode of a very long-lasting migraine attack will not cause MIH. The type of excessive use we are talking about involves taking pain relievers regularly over weeks – even years, for some people. Patients describe their underlying, almost constant headache as 'dull', 'sickly' and 'a feeling of pressure'. They differentiate the type of daily head pain from their typical, more severe migraine attacks (which continue to occur on occasion). The underlying headache is often present on waking in the morning, or comes on soon after getting out of bed, as the sufferer faces the ordinary challenges of his or her day. Other symptoms such as forgetfulness, difficulty concentrating, restlessness and nausea may accompany the headache. The need for pain relievers usually increases over time, and the sufferer may find that an escalation in strength of the preparation is necessary (many graduate to the use of preparations containing codeine quite quickly). Although the pain relievers do not offer anywhere near complete relief, the sufferer continues to take them, largely out of fear that a full-blown attack will ensue if he or she doesn't 'get ahead' of the pain. Indeed, when the overuse of pain relievers is stopped, the headache will *temporarily* get worse. But this temporary worsening must be looked upon as short-term pain for long-term gain as the medication works its way out of the body's system. Once

---

MIH warning signs

1. Daily, or almost daily, headache.
2. Symptoms may also include nausea, forgetfulness and/or restlessness.
3. Headache present on waking, may wake sufferer from sleep or may be brought on through the smallest physical or intellectual effort.
4. Daily, or almost daily, use of pain relievers.
5. Increasing need for pain relievers.
6. Headache temporarily worsens if use of pain reliever stopped.
7. Preventive medications ineffective until overuse of pain relievers is stopped.

the person is over the hump, the headaches will dramatically improve. *The only way to stop MIH is to stop the overuse of the offending medication.* It's as simple as that, although the action of stopping is much more challenging. The effort put forth towards breaking the rebound cycle will probably be rewarded by an end to the low-lying, sickly pain. Preventive medications prescribed to reduce the number of headaches experienced will be ineffective unless the rebound-causing medication is stopped.

Those with medication-induced headache must realize they are not alone. People caught in the vicious cycle of overuse are neither 'bad' nor 'addicts'. Although studies have not yet been conducted to determine scientifically the number of people with MIH, the incidence is believed to be alarmingly high. At public forums on migraine, almost all participants raise their hands when asked if they believe that there is some element of MIH involved with their migraine. This problem is of paramount concern to headache experts world-wide.

Stopping the use of the offending pain relievers or ergotamines is essential in the treatment of MIH. Studies have shown that stopping the medication will lead to a profound reduction in headaches. With much willpower, some people may be able to stop cold turkey. Others will be advised by their doctors to reduce their intake slowly, for example, by cutting down the use of pain-relieving medication at a rate of 10–20 per cent each week. But no matter how the pills are stopped, the headaches will likely get worse before they get better, as the body's system rights itself. The first month is the hardest. Tomorrow will be a better day, and next month will be better than this month! If the overuse isn't stopped now, the head pain and other symptoms will only continue to get worse.

To stop reaching for the pill bottle – which for some has become a reflex response – various strategies can be tried. At the first twinge, some people take a break to stretch out cramped legs and tense muscles in the neck, upper back and shoulder area. Taking a few deep breaths and a brisk walk is another good idea. A cup of hot tea, or a cold beverage if preferred, will provide a needed break. Non-drug strategies such as biofeedback or relaxation techniques are an important addition to therapy for many. Rubbing the temples with Tiger Balm, a Chinese ointment found in many pharmacies, or putting an icepack on the back of the neck, can provide added comfort. Mild or moderate headache pain should no longer be treated with medication, although use of some medications will be okayed by the doctor in cases of severe attacks.

Keeping a positive attitude during the time spent getting off the rebound-causing medication is very important. Some imagine the period during which they get off painkillers as recovery time from surgery, and prepare for it by trying to minimize the time devoted to unnecessary obligations and to maximize the time available for pampering themselves. Others have employed strategies similar to those used in trying to quit smoking, or adhering to a slimming programme. Eliciting the support of family and close friends will be critical. They can be strong allies if properly educated about MIH and the effort involved in breaking the cycle of overuse.

If, however, treatment with symptomatic medication has involved taking a lot of prescription drugs containing codeine, narcotics or tranquillizers, it may be necessary to taper off under a doctor's supervision. Rarely, tapering off will involve admission to hospital so that special medications (such as dihydroergotamine) that can't usually be administered in the outpatient setting can be implemented to help break the cycle of resistant rebound or to manage withdrawal reactions. However, most people will be able to break the cycle of overuse at home.

A headache journal or diary is an essential tool for all seeking to reduce the use of pain relievers. These records will measure progress, which may seem slow at first but will become obvious when written down and examined over time. It is important to make a baseline recording (a notation of normal consumption) for a couple of weeks before the pain relievers are reduced. From there, many people see a rise in headaches as the pills are taken away, followed by a gradual improvement. Many types of journals have been designed and implemented throughout the years, but they need not be elaborate. It may be simplest to purchase a month-at-a-glance wall calendar with large squares for each day to allow enough room to record the following information:

- days (hours) with headache
- severity of headache (from mild to very severe)
- other symptoms experienced
- medication taken
- suspected triggers
- for women, days of menstrual period.

Keeping such a journal can help sufferers learn a great deal about their headache, headache triggers and use of medication. It's better to examine recorded fact than to rely on memory, which may overlook the subtleties.

When reducing the intake of pain relievers, always remember that one study on the subject revealed that almost 50 per cent of chronic daily rebound headaches will go away in a few weeks once the overuse of analgesics or ergotamines is stopped, even if no other treatment is implemented.

The next step in combating the rebound effect may involve the use of appropriate preventive medications to correct the underlying problem in brain chemistry. After all, the underlying problem that started the cycle of overuse is still there! Specific preventive medications are discussed in Chapter 8. If preventive therapy is considered, many doctors will start by trying an antidepressant medication first (not because the patient is depressed, but because antidepressants have an anti-headache property). Other doctors will suggest trying a beta blocker or calcium-channel blocker. In any case, it is very important to realize that preventive medications will work only after use of the rebound-causing medication is stopped.

Part of the new treatment may include the judicious, infrequent use of pain relievers for severe attacks, but not until the sufferer is out of the woods as far as overuse goes. More commonly, the doctor may prescribe non-narcotic anti-inflammatory or migraine-specific medication to help break the cycle of medication-induced headache and to address the symptoms of any breakthrough attacks that occur while on the preventive regime. Limits and conditions must be decided upon by doctor and patient concerning the use of any symptomatic medication to prevent a relapse into rebound.

Managing rebound involves a permanent change in behaviour. The fear of attacks must be overcome through good migraine management rather than through medicating every twinge of pain. Regular exercise to boost the body's production of endorphins is critical in reducing headaches (brisk walking is an excellent choice). Avoiding identified migraine triggers, using biofeedback and adopting other non-drug strategies described in Chapter 12 may also be considered part of a treatment plan.

Once a programme is put in place, you should stay in

Seven steps to breaking the cycle of rebound

1. Recognize the problem.
2. Learn about the negative effects of the overuse of pain relievers and what the alternatives are.
3. Stop the medication(s) causing the rebound.
4. Consider medications and/or non-drug strategies to help break the cycle of rebound headaches.
5. Consider medications and/or non-drug strategies to prevent further attacks.
6. Consider medications and/or non-drug strategies to deal with any breakthrough migraine attacks that occur after the cycle of rebound is broken.
7. Stay in touch with the doctor.

---

touch with your doctor in order that progress can be monitored and any necessary adjustments to treatment can be made. Dose adjustments and medication changes are almost always necessary.

Finally, it's important to point out once again that some people will experience an evolution of their migraine into a daily headache disorder in which overuse of medication is *not* a factor. Whether medication is implicated or not, it is essential to work closely with a doctor who is knowledgeable about daily headache.

Cluster headache

Cluster headache is five times more common in men than in women. It affects less than 1 per cent of the population and, unlike migraine, does not tend to run in families. It can occur at any age, but seems to occur more frequently in men aged twenty to forty years.

Cluster headaches are not migraine attacks. Cluster headache should not be referred to as 'cluster migraine'. Even though the symptoms of cluster headache are distinctly different from those of migraine and are fairly easily recognized, many people who have migraine attacks in periods of fits and starts are wrongly told that they suffer from 'cluster'. If you have any doubt about your diagnosis, this section may help clarify it for you.

Although cluster headache sits alone in its diagnostic category, like migraine it results from a biological disorder that affects blood flow and nerve transmission in the body's central nervous system. 'Cluster' derives its name from the nature of the pain it causes. Attacks are grouped in a series lasting for weeks or months (so-called cluster periods) separated by pain-free periods of months or years (however, about 10 per cent of cluster sufferers have chronic attacks that continue without remission). Often the cluster period returns at the same time each year (in many cases, during the months in which the number of hours of sunlight undergoes significant change, owing to the role of the light-sensitive hypothalamus in the brain). The characteristic pain of cluster headache arrives in short, intensely severe bursts, usually lasting from thirty to forty-five minutes, and rarely lasting longer than four hours. The severe pain is often described as 'a hot poker' penetrating one eye and is experienced from once every other day up to eight times daily. The side of the head on which the pain is felt can vary between attacks, but it almost never occurs on both sides at the same time. During an attack, a sufferer may also experience on the painful side of his or her head:

- eye redness and tearing
- nasal congestion
- running from the nostril
- forehead and facial sweating

- constriction of the pupil
- drooping of the eyelid
- swelling of the eyelid.

The pain is so intense that the sufferer is often unable to stay still, and may pace uncontrollably, unlike the migraine sufferer, who often finds relief by lying quietly. The attacks tend to occur at the same time each day, often waking the sufferer from a stage of sleep known as REM (rapid eye movement) sleep. Although the cause of cluster headache is not fully understood, it may be that the attacks occur in response to the body's chemical changes associated with sleep, or perhaps it, too, is related to the hypothalamus's internal clock. A study published in the *Lancet* in 2000 revealed low levels of the hormone melatonin in cluster patients. Another explanation probes the theory of inflammation of an area behind the face called the 'cavernous sinus', while work done by Professor Peter Goadsby has revealed structural differences in the brains of cluster sufferers.

Clinical observation over the years has led some researchers to note that many (but not all) cluster sufferers share some characteristics:

- ruddy complexion
- multi-furrowed thick skin (*peau d'orange* or skin somewhat like orange peel)
- tendency to smoke cigarettes or drink alcohol
- 20 per cent incidence of a history of peptic ulcer.

During the cluster period, anything that causes the enlargement of blood vessels may trigger an attack. Alcohol must be avoided during this time. A food additive known as MSG (monosodium glutamate), often added to fast foods and prepared foods, must also be avoided. Some sufferers also report that changes in altitude and air travel, as well as strong sunlight, changes in sleep patterns and the 'come-down' period from stress, are potential triggers of cluster attacks. However, during the period between clusters, nothing will trigger an attack. Since smoking may be connected to cluster, it is advisable for the sufferer to quit.

Treatment becomes an urgent need once the cluster headache begins. Often a referral to a neurologist will be quickly made. Doctors find they often consider intervention using medical treatments. One treatment that is gaining in popularity is breathing pure oxygen from a tank at the onset of an attack. An oxygen tank can be set up where the person usually experiences the attacks (often next to the bed). It is important that the mask fits tightly and has no side vents. The dial should be set at 7 litres per minute, and the sufferer should sit with his or her upper body and head leaning forward. Often relief comes within fifteen minutes.

Another treatment sometimes used involves the use of lidocaine nosedrops during a cluster attack. Usually 1 millilitre of 4 per cent lidocaine (a solution used as a topical anaesthetic) is dropped into the nostril on the affected side while the sufferer lies on his or her back with the head extended and tipped over the edge of the bed, sofa or table.

Painkillers used to treat attacks already in progress often do not work rapidly enough to stop the pain of a cluster headache. By the time the medication begins to work, the cluster attack has usually subsided on its own. Since the attacks occur frequently during the cluster period, it is usually not advisable to take narcotic painkillers (even if they help) as often as would be required. Other medications that contain the blood-vessel constrictor ergotamine may be helpful to some, but must not be used more often than prescribed, owing to the potential negative effects of overuse. A group of medications that appears to be promising in research, but is not yet approved for use in cluster by the regulatory bodies, is the triptans – especially sumatriptan by injection, as it works fastest. More traditionally, however, doctors will prescribe preventive medications such as methysergide, chlorpromazine, lithium, or verapamil at the early signs of a cluster period (more information on all medications is provided in Chapter 8). The anti-epileptic medication topiramate is currently being studied for cluster 'prevention'. Steroids such as prednisotone (not the body-building type) and non-steroidal anti-inflammatories, as well as medications that desensitize the patient to histamine, have also been tried more traditionally for treatment of acute attacks. As well, freezing local nerves with injections (see 'Post-traumatic Headache', below) may provide temporary relief.

In rare chronic cases of cluster headache that is resistant to all therapies, surgery may be considered. Using microwaves, the surgeon operates on the fifth cranial (trigeminal) nerve ganglion. 'Radiofrequency lesions' made through the unbroken skin deaden the nerve in a procedure called 'percutaneous trigeminal rhizotomy'. Side effects can result, such as permanent loss of sensation or a loss of corneal reflex in the eye (which can result in corneal infection or ulceration). The procedure is not guaranteed to be effective (in one doctor's opinion, it is effective in two out of three patients). In one case, the pain recurred on the sufferer's opposite side three days after surgery. Nevertheless, in some circumstances a patient may wish to examine the options and weigh the pros and cons of this treatment with a knowledgeable and experienced practitioner.

Chronic paroxysmal hemicrania

Chronic paroxysmal hemicrania (CPH) is similar to cluster headache, although, whereas cluster mainly affects men, CPH affects mainly women. The painful attacks of CPH are shorter (lasting 2 to 45 minutes, unlike cluster, which usually lasts from 30 to 45 minutes or more) and more frequent. The good news is that these attacks can almost always be stopped by taking the prescription non-steroidal anti-inflammatory indomethacin.

Hemicrania continua

Although not validated by the International Headache Society, hemicrania continua (or hemicrania continuat) is believed by many experts to be a rare headache disorder that involves a continuous mild-to-moderate form of headache, with additional bouts of severe pain lasting from minutes to days. The spikes of pain may have a quality similar to that of a cluster headache. It is almost always completely controlled by the use of indomethacin.

Post-traumatic headache

Post-traumatic headache occurs after a head injury. This type of headache can follow even the mildest head injury, and often no evidence of physical damage to the brain or surrounding structures shows up on a CAT or MRI scan. Although post-traumatic headache is not universally recognized to be directly related to migraine, its actual cause is still unknown and debated. Some doctors use the term 'cervicogenic headache' to describe headaches that are believed to be caused by structural problems within the neck, many of which are caused by accidents. Cervicogenic headache differs from migraine in that such symptoms as nausea, vomiting, sensitivity to light and sensitivity to sound are usually less intense. The pain of a cervicogenic headache tends to start in the neck, then spread forward over the back of the head to the front. Neck mobility is often reduced and pain may result when the neck is moved certain ways. As well, one-sided shoulder and/or arm pain may be present. Pain can often be produced when the doctor presses the back of the scalp above what is called the 'greater occipital nerve'.

In the past, post-traumatic headache that was not associated with obvious physical damage was believed to be solely psychological in nature. Many experts believed that the symptoms were 'put on' in an effort to obtain financial compensation from insurance companies. Others felt it was a psychosomatic reaction to the frightening accident. In *bona fide* cases, however, nothing could be farther from the truth. The severe and debilitating symptoms of post-traumatic headache can include headaches of either migrainous or a related type, memory loss, dizziness, difficulty with concentration, decreased sexual desire and in some cases personality changes, which can include sudden bursts of anger. A biological mechanism generates these symptoms. It stands to reason that treatment of the effects of such dramatic symptoms may involve psychotherapy, but the problem is certainly not psychological.

Discussion of the treatment of post-traumatic headache is too lengthy for this book; however, it usually follows a 'multidisciplinary' approach involving several different types of treatment and/or care-givers working together. It is important in the context of this book to mention that the changes in the underlying mechanism within the brain of someone suffering from post-traumatic headache may involve some of the elements of migraine, and therefore some of the treatments for post-traumatic headache and migraine may overlap.

The treatment of post-traumatic, or cervicogenic, headache may include any combination of physiotherapy, cervical manipulations by trained physicians, biofeedback, relaxation training, counselling, special exercises and the use of traditional medications. Nerve blocks, which involve freezing certain large nerves through injections of local anaesthetic which may or may not be mixed with steroids to reduce inflammation, may bring temporary relief to some sufferers. These nerve blocks may also be used for the treatment of migraine with or without aura, but are significantly more effective in treating cervicogenic headache. Injections may be given into the scalp to freeze the greater occipital nerve and its branches, or into the area above the eyebrow to freeze the supraorbital nerve.

Sinus headache

Recurrent sinus headaches are relatively rare. Many people who think they have sinus headache are actually suffering from another form of headache or from migraine. Migraine sufferers can experience watery eyes or a stuffy or runny nose during their attacks, owing to a histamine response associated with the disorder. Sinus infections can cause pain in the face and adjacent areas of the head, but true sinus infections are almost always accompanied by fever, nasal congestion and a general feeling of illness which may be more severe than the pain itself. The false belief that one suffers from sinus headache rather than migraine may be supported by the fact that many non-prescription sinus medications may help with the pain. In fact, migraine sufferers often obtain a measure of temporary relief from these products, which can contain pain relievers. The antihistamine component of these medications may also help with the symptoms of migraine. However, non-prescription preparations are rarely fully effective and may cause a worsening of the headache disorder through the rebound effect. Advertising for such products may lead people to believe that they have so-called sinus headache when in fact they have another type of headache disorder – possibly even migraine.

Allergic headache

Some people think their headaches are caused by allergies. The true allergy headache, like the sinus headache, is relatively rare. In fact, it is more common for the allergy sufferer to also experience tension-type or migraine headache. Often the confusion results from a situation in which a particular food is capable of producing headache in an individual. The headache is then mistakenly interpreted as being an *allergic* response. In fact, it is likely that the person is a migraine sufferer, and that the chemical content of the food or beverage consumed has triggered a *migrainous* response.

Eyestrain headache

In order to avoid eyestrain headache, it is important to take regular breaks from tedious work or activities that involve visual concentration. Regular eye examinations are important. If your vision is impaired, always make sure that your glasses are clean and not heavily scratched, and that the lenses match your most recent prescription. Contact-lens wearers must fastidiously follow cleaning and storage directions. (See Chapter 7 for more on eyestrain as a migraine trigger in the workplace.)

Benign exertional headache

Benign exertional headache is brought on by very intense physical exercise. Weightlifters are the group most likely to suffer from this type of headache, particularly if they suffer other types of headaches such as migraine. People who, for occupational or other reasons, must continue intense physical strain should see their doctor. Some may find relief by taking anti-inflammatories or medications that constrict blood vessels before participating in such demanding activities.

Sex headache

As the name implies, these headaches are brought on by sexual activities that result in orgasm (including masturbation). The headache usually starts as a dull ache, then intensifies at orgasm. The head pain can last from a few minutes to several hours. This type of headache is sometimes experienced by people with migraine. However, the sudden development of an incapacitating headache with orgasm could also be the ominous sign of a life-threatening problem, and should be checked out at the emergency department immediately.

Ice-cream headache

Many migraine sufferers can recall experiencing headache from eating ice cream early in childhood, long before their migraine was ever diagnosed. Ice-cream headache is thought by many to be a precursor to migraine. The pain is short-lived but intense, and occurs when one eats very cold food, such as ice cream. Ice-cream headache is often felt in the area behind the eyes. The treatment is instinctive – eat ice cream slowly, in small amounts.

Idiopathic stabbing headache

Many migraine sufferers have experienced 'ice-pick' pains, and perhaps have come to ignore them because they go away so quickly. Others have them so often that they become bothersome. Although 'ice-pick' pains occur in people who don't get migraine, they are more common among migraineurs. The pain feels as though an ice pick is stabbing into the head, commonly in the area of the head where migraine pain is usually felt. It lasts only a fraction of a second and can occur as a single stab or a series of them. They are usually felt more often when a migraine attack is in progress. If treatment is necessary, the prescription anti-inflammatory drug indomethacin is often effective.

Substance-abuse headaches and hangovers

Anyone suffering from any type of recurring headache should avoid alcoholic beverages. Alcohol can cause headaches in people who don't even have a headache disorder!

Alcohol acts to dilate (widen) blood vessels, as is apparent from the red facial complexion of drinkers once they've had a few. The dilation also occurs in the blood vessels surrounding the brain – the same vessels involved in a migraine attack. The chemicals that cause this dilation are found in higher amounts in 'coloured' alcohols such as red wine, Scotch, rum and beer. (Red wine is almost always off-limits for headache sufferers.)

Alcohol also causes the body's blood-sugar level to be thrown off. When a drink is taken, the blood-sugar level rises rapidly, then very quickly plummets. Alcohols with a high sugar content (such as liqueurs) will worsen this problem. Using a soft drink that contains sugar as a 'mixer' may add to the problem, but some headache sufferers report trouble even with the sugar substitutes used in diet version (notably aspartame). Using water, soda water or vegetable juice as a 'mixer' may help. The drop in blood sugar that results after drinking alcohol works in tandem with the alcohol-dilated blood vessels as an additional headache trigger. The blood-sugar levels will endure an even faster and more dramatic roller-coaster ride if the alcohol is ingested on an empty stomach.

Hangovers are caused by these same mechanisms. In addition, alcohol causes dehydration as it interferes with the normal production of a hormone which regulates the body's fluid level. Once this hormone is depleted, excess water is lost from the body in the form of urine. The brain's fluid level is also depleted in the process and the brain and nerve tissue cry out in pain as a result. This process also happens in people who don't suffer from a headache disorder. Some drinkers attempt to restore the fluid lost by drinking one glass of water for each alcoholic beverage consumed throughout the evening and then having two full glasses of water before going to bed. Hangovers may occur more readily in drinkers who are headache sufferers, and can occur in headache-prone people who have ingested small amounts of alcohol.

Many drugs, such as cocaine, can produce headache. As we have seen in rebound headache, withdrawal from drugs can also result in head pain. The 'hair of the dog that bit you' principle subscribed to by heavy drinkers, in which they start the morning off with a drink to get over their hangover, works largely by correcting the substance-withdrawal symptoms.

One drug that is reported by some migraine sufferers to have the capacity to alleviate attacks is marijuana. This knowledge is not new, by any means. William Gowers, an eminent physician of the late 1800s, recommended smoking Indian hemp for the relief of migraine attacks. Marijuana, hashish and hash oil are all products of the hemp plant, *Cannabis sativa*. Although the chief ingredient in marijuana, delta-9-tetrahydrocannabinol (THC), has been studied for the treatment of disorders such as multiple sclerosis (MS), chronic pain conditions, glaucoma and nausea caused by chemotherapy, there are no generally accepted medical uses for it today. (Studies are in progress, but not with regard to migraine.) Cannabis is also, of course, currently strictly legislated, and penalties for possession can include fines and imprisonment. Animal experiments have shown that high doses of cannabis can cause chromosome damage, low levels of the male sex hormone and reduced defences against infection and brain damage.

Migraine sufferers who spend an evening out at a dance club, bar or local pub may develop a headache – even if they don't consume alcohol! The flashing lights and loud noise in a club can send heads throbbing. Cigarette smoke is also a big culprit. Both first- and secondhand cigarette smoke are a problem for sufferers of benign headache disorders, and nowhere is secondhand smoke thicker than in a bar. Although nicotine constricts blood vessels, it doesn't seem to have a therapeutic effect on migraine sufferers. The other toxic chemicals in the smoke seem to override any beneficial effects. One study showed that, by eliminating triggers and quitting smoking, 53 per cent of ex-smokers became headache free. In contrast, only 13 per cent of non-smokers became headache free when they eliminated dietary triggers. The extra gains made by the smokers seemed to result from kicking the habit.

Lupus headaches

Systemic lupus erythematosus is a disorder that is usually believed to be quite separate and distinct from migraine. However, the symptoms of lupus may mimic migraine, making the diagnosis tricky in some instances. In addition, sufferers of lupus are more likely to suffer from migraine than are members of the general population. The symptoms of lupus itself may include a form of non-migrainous headache. Treatment for the symptoms of lupus often results in a reduction of both migraine and non-migraine headaches.

Other types of benign headaches

Other types of non-life-threatening headache syndromes include *external compression headache* (formerly called 'swim-goggle headache'), which results from continued pressure on the nerves of the scalp, and *benign cough headache*, which can be brought on by coughing in an otherwise totally healthy person. See Chapter 7 for a discussion of temporomandibular (joint) disorder – known as TMD or TMJ.

Life-threatening types of headache

Fortunately, the vast majority of headache sufferers will not be diagnosed with what we all fear – a life-threatening problem. Headaches caused by brain tumours are very rare. Indeed, it is almost unheard of that the first symptom of a brain tumor is headache. Usually the first symptoms of a tumour involve visual problems or other neurological symptoms.

It is rare that a physician will order sophisticated tests to aid in the diagnosis of your benign headache problem, as such tests are seldom necessary. However, despite the low incidence of life-threatening problems, from time to time doctors order specific tests to rule out ominous causes of headache. If you are scheduled for one or some of these tests, don't think the worst, and try not to jump to conclusions.

Headaches with fever

Headaches that occur in tandem with a fever are usually not serious. The common cold, flu, or other run-of-the-mill viruses can cause fever and headache. Usually the symptoms of these illnesses can be relieved with bed rest and non-prescription medications like paracetamol to bring the fever down and to relieve the headache pain. When headache accompanies these common viral illnesses, it is merely an annoyance. Fever itself can cause headache. Ear infection is a relatively common cause of fever in children and headache can also be present with the infection. Migraine sufferers often find that their attacks can be triggered by another illness, often as the other illness is 'on its way out'. Many report that, just as they are getting over a bout of cold or flu, they are stricken with a full-blown migraine.

However, fevers can accompany headache as part of a serious illness. Meningitis is suspected when the headache is accompanied by fever, stiff neck, nausea, vomiting and a general feeling of weakness and unwellness. Although rare, encephalitis is suspected if confusion, seizures and extreme drowsiness are present along with fever and headache.

Headache caused by malformations of blood vessels

Certain types of structural malformations of blood vessels in the head can cause serious complications. As well, aneurysms (ballooning of blood vessels) in the head can rupture, causing bleeding within the closed vault of the skull. This, in turn, causes pressure on the brain, which can result in a sudden headache followed by loss of consciousness. A ruptured aneurysm – thankfully rare – is very serious. The hallmark symptom of a ruptured aneurysm is the sudden onset (like a thunderclap) of a headache worse than any experienced previously. It may come on while the person is at rest, or during heavy exertion (including during sexual activity). Immediate emergency care is required if such a headache occurs, particularly if it is accompanied by behavioural or memory changes, a decreased level of consciousness or seizure.

Headache caused by lesions

Although rarely found to be the cause of recurring headache, growths, abscesses, tumours, cysts and strokes can cause head pain. Headache is not usually the first symptom of these potentially life-threatening problems. Tumours, for instance, must usually be quite large before they are capable of pressing on pain-sensitive nerve endings. Usually the sufferer notices behavioural or memory changes and neurological symptoms such as difficulty with balance and walking, and visual impairment, long before any pain is felt. In stroke, the patient detects a one-sided weakness as a first symptom, or visual or sensory loss.

If the headache is caused by an underlying lesion, it does not tend to wax and wane – that is, it doesn't tend to worsen and get better, then worsen again. The head pain will be relatively constant and, without treatment, will likely steadily worsen over time. The head pain of a growth in the brain or its immediate surroundings may be worse upon rising in the morning. People who have experienced headaches for years and years usually need not fear that their pain is being caused by a tumour; tumours are very likely to increase in size over time, and those who have them notice a deterioration in health without medical intervention.

However, since a slight chance does exist that the headache may be caused by an underlying lesion, proper diagnosis by a doctor is essential. It is of particular importance in the older population, as the chance of life-threatening problems developing increases slightly with age.

Anyone of any age who experiences a new type of headache, a headache accompanied by unusual symptoms, or a headache that is worse than any previously experienced – particularly if it comes on suddenly – should check with a doctor or emergency department without delay.

4
Women and Migraine:
The Hormonal Influence

Around the world, two to three times as many women suffer from migraine as men. The impact of migraine on women's health is substantial. In a survey reported by the Genesis Research Foundation, the biggest health fears expressed by women were breast, ovarian and other cancers; heart disease; and road accidents. The non-life-threatening issues of most concern to women included arthritis and *chronic headaches*.

Books and articles written as late as 1991 incorrectly blame the stressful dual roles women play as both home-makers and career people for this increased incidence. This false belief unnecessarily complicates migraine management and, in many cases, it is to blame for migraine not being taken seriously.

The central reason why most migraine sufferers are women is biological – namely, the influence of female hormones. Consider this: twice as many young boys suffer from migraine as do young girls, but at puberty this ratio reverses and continues through adult life.

One study showed that migraine hits hardest women between the ages of 25 and 44. In another study, 25 per cent of female migraine sufferers had one or more attacks per week and 35 per cent had one to three *severe* attacks per month. And another study showed that 78 per cent of migraine sufferers reported that their normal routine was affected during their last attack.

Recently it has been recognized that migraine may actually follow a standard pattern in the life of many women. The following typical life history may unfold for many, but certainly not all, women who suffer from migraine:

Cathy Smith's mother remembers experiencing headaches during high school on the first day of her period. Back in those days, no one spoke much of 'feminine afflictions', so she struggled through those days in silence. She would have the odd headache at other times during the month as well, but fortunately they usually went away after she slept for a few hours.

When Cathy's mother married, although she still got headaches, they were infrequent. When she was pregnant, however, her headaches occurred more frequently for the first three months or so. She also thought they were more severe, but couldn't be sure if she thought so simply because she couldn't 'catch' them with the pain relievers she was able to take when not pregnant. Fortunately, by the time she entered the fourth month of each pregnancy, her headaches virtually disappeared. However, all good things must come to an end and Cathy's mother would experience severe headaches immediately after giving birth. It was during a really bad attack while in hospital after having her second child that Cathy's mother was diagnosed by her doctor as suffering from migraine. That attack was preceded by a blank spot before her eyes that her doctor explained was the warning sign, or aura, of a migraine attack.

During Cathy's mother's thirties and forties, she continued to suffer from full-blown migraine attacks (some with aura), both with her periods and at other times. Her use of medication to cope with the pain and to 'get ahead' of the pain increased. In addition to her usual attacks, she also developed an almost constant low-lying headache. Some days were worse than others, although she could usually continue with her day despite the discomfort.

During menopause, this headache pattern continued to worsen. It wasn't until Cathy's mother was fully through menopause that her headaches disappeared. She is still left with a remnant in the form of visual disturbances. Thankfully, the migraine pain no longer follows the aura.

It is not surprising that Cathy's mother suffered from migraine. A 1990 study showed that 66 per cent of migraine sufferers have a close blood relative who also suffers, and 53 per cent of those relatives are mothers.

Changes in the balance between the hormones oestrogen and progesterone influence the higher incidence of migraine in women. For reasons not yet understood, migraine can be triggered by a low oestrogen level in some women (such as right before a menstrual period or right after childbirth) and a high oestrogen level in other women (such as when taking the birth-control pill or hormone-replacement therapy).

Menstrual migraine

A study showed that, although more than 50 per cent of English women report that their migraine is linked to menstrual periods, only 10 per cent experience migraines only during their periods (true menstrual migraine), and 35 per cent have migraines that are related to their periods but also at other times as well. Other factors also relate migraine to the menstrual period. Around the time of the period, there is a decrease in the body's level of endorphins (naturally occurring painkillers). As well, migraine is associated with fluid retention, as is menstruation.

Special considerations in the treatment of menstrual migraine

After establishing a relationship between migraine and menstrual periods from the evidence in a headache diary, and after instituting the 'usual' strategies for the treatment of migraine, such as eliminating controllable triggers and using symptomatic medications to help control any attacks that occur, doctors may suggest the preventive treatment of menstrual migraine with medication taken around the time of the period. Whereas regular preventive drug therapy involves taking medication every day, menstrual-migraine medication is taken from about three days before the period is due to begin until three or four days after the first day of menstruation. If the periods are irregular, it may not be possible to consider this option, since predicting when the next period is due is essential. So, traditional daily use of preventives may be chosen instead. However, if the doctor and patient decide to try 'perimenstrual prophylaxis', or the use of preventive medications only around the time of the period, medications that block the production of prostaglandins may be tried. Prostaglandins are pain-producing substances that are released from the uterus around the time of the period. Since their release is believed to trigger migraine in some (and is the culprit behind menstrual cramps as well), it makes sense to try to block their production. Non-steroidal anti-inflammatory medications used for this purpose may include mefenamic acid, naproxen or ibuprofen. Researchers are now examining the use of oestrogen patches around the time of the period to stop the drop in oestrogen level believed to act as a migraine trigger. Others are studying the use of a 1-milligram dose of naratriptan (a migraine-specific agent) for the prevention of menstrual migraine.

Other possible therapies for menstrual migraine target the reduction of premenstrual syndrome (PMS). If symptoms of PMS, such as irritability, fluid retention, breast tenderness or abdominal bloating are present, measures such as limiting salt intake, avoiding alcoholic beverages and beverages containing caffeine and participating in regular exercise may help with both the PMS and the migraine. Magnesium has also been examined as a supplement to reduce migraines (see Chapter 12, 'Complementary Therapies').

Back in the 1960s it was the practice in some areas to perform a radical or total hysterectomy on women suffering from hormone related migraine. The theory was simple: remove the offending hormones, stop the migraine. Although some women did benefit, others did not, and some actually got worse. Since this treatment involves major abdominal surgery and propels the system into instant menopause, exposing women to other health risks associated with early menopause such as heart disease and osteoporosis, it cannot be recommended as a treatment for migraine. Today, however, if it is considered necessary to interrupt the effects of female hormones, doctors can initiate a trial of a medication such as danazol or nafarelin acetate, which will temporarily shut down ovarian function, mimicking the effects that surgical removal of the ovaries would have. Evaluation may be made over a longer period after the administration of a long-lasting injection of medications such as leuprolide acetate. A woman considering medications to shut down ovarian function may wish to consult her own neurologist and gynaecologist when weighing up the potential benefits against the potential risks of therapy. This type of drug treatment is considered only after traditional therapies have been tried without success. Surgical removal of the ovaries (oophorectomy) is almost never considered.

The use of the birth-control pill or hormone-replacement therapy must be considered on an individual basis; either treatment will make some people worse, others better, and have no effect at all on still others, since hormones are not the root cause of all migraine in women.

Migraine and the birth-control pill

If the birth-control pill is prescribed, using the lowest dose possible is probably a good idea. Women who are affected by menstrually related migraine may find that their attacks are more likely to occur during the week in the pill cycle in which no pills (or placebos) are taken. Over the years, there has been much discussion among doctors about the use of the birth-control pill by women who suffer from migraine. Some doctors will advise against its use in all types of migraine. Other doctors will prescribe the pill to migraine sufferers, but monitor them for any increase in the quantity or severity of migraines experienced. Use of the pill will be discontinued if it worsens migraine. Many doctors agree, however, that women who regularly experience migraine with aura (other than typical visual auras) should avoid the birth-control pill altogether and opt for other effective methods of contraception. The rationale is that the combination of migraine with aura and the use of the pill may slightly raise the patient's risk of permanent damage resulting from a stroke that reduces blood flow to areas of the brain. Some doctors feel the low-dose birth-control pills are much less likely to cause problems than older varieties of the pill, which contained much higher hormone levels. If a woman with migraine is considering taking the birth-control pill, she should discuss the benefits as well as the risks involved and come to an informed decision with the help of her doctor. One thing is certain, however, about the use of the birth-control pill: the combination of taking the pill and smoking cigarettes greatly increases a woman's risk of stroke at any age. For a woman who gets migraine, takes the pill and smokes, there is even more risk.

Migraine and hormone-replacement therapy

Hormone-replacement therapy (HRT) is given to some women to minimize health risks associated with the post-menopausal period and to treat symptoms such as hot flushes and mood swings. In the past, HRT was often prescribed in a cycle of 21 days on, 7 days off, in an attempt to mimic the body's natural production of oestrogen. However, women who took oestrogen cyclically often had their menopausal symptoms return during the seven days off and women with migraine tended to have more headaches during the same seven days. More recently, oestrogen has often been given daily through a skin patch or in tablet form in order to avoid the problems that occur during the seven days without oestrogen. Unless the woman taking hormone-replacement therapy has had a hysterectomy, she will be prescribed a progesterone hormone as well (usually in pill form). The progesterone will create a menstrual period and help to protect against cancer of the uterus. The progesterone is not likely to affect migraine because oestrogen is the hormone believed to play the major role in migraine. Currently there is little information on how headache is affected by natural plant hormones or by the newer selective agent raloxifene (an oestrogen receptor modulator).

Some women taking hormone replacements will actually feel better as the hormonal fluctuations of menopause are brought under control. Others will not notice any change in their migraine pattern if hormone-replacement therapy is prescribed for medical reasons during the menopause. Unfortunately, others will find their headaches worsen. Any woman who is taking hormone-replacement therapy, or considering it, must discuss her personal case with her own doctor.

Migraine in pregnancy

Sufferers of severe or frequent migraine face additional considerations when planning a family. 'Who will help with the baby if I get an attack?' and 'What will I do if I can't take medication for any attacks I have when I'm pregnant?' are common concerns of potential mothers-to-be who get migraine. These are valid concerns and must be thought through quite carefully.

Nature often seems to bring an exaggerated state of health to many pregnant women. For some women with migraine, the last 6 months of pregnancy may be a period when they have never felt better. Migraine tends to improve during pregnancy more often in women whose migraines were previously associated with their menstrual periods. Other women will not be so lucky, and will continue to have migraine attacks throughout their pregnancy. A very few report that their symptoms actually worsen. Migraine can begin for the very first time during pregnancy, especially during the first three months. The treatment of migraine in pregnant women presents a special challenge. The use of medication becomes very limited because not much is known about how teratogenic (damaging to the foetus) many of these drugs may be. For this reason, non-drug treatment strategies become even more important to research and employ diligently. Almost all women with migraine are likely to experience one or more attacks during the first three to four months of pregnancy, so investigating the non-drug options before trying to become pregnant is a good idea.

Pregnant women seeking to gain control over their migraines must be extra careful to eat healthy foods and get proper rest. Regular exercise in pregnancy is good for the prevention of headaches. If migraine occurs, applying cold packs (or heat packs, if preferred) and climbing into bed may provide comfort. Some doctors may okay the infrequent use of paracetamol and may administer pethidine during very severe attacks. Some medications are absolutely contraindicated during pregnancy, while others are allowed. Before taking medications, the woman must discuss the potential risks to the foetus with her doctor, and come to an informed decision about the ratio of risks to benefits. Note that if there are risks, they are often greatest in the first three months.

Expectant mothers should take comfort in knowing that, although they may still get migraine, they do not have an increased risk of complications associated with their pregnancy. It is also reassuring to know that children born to women who suffer from migraine while pregnant do not show any increased incidence of birth defects.

As the anticipated moment of delivery grows closer, women usually begin to think about pain control during the delivery. The use of epidural anaesthesia during delivery is quite common, especially for first-time deliveries. The epidural involves the insertion of a needle into the epidural space around the spinal cord in the lower back. Local anaesthetic, narcotics or both are injected into the epidural space through a small catheter that is often left in place, allowing the anaesthetist to 'top up' the medication later on, if necessary. Since the epidural may be associated with a headache after it is removed, migraine sufferers are sometimes concerned about agreeing to an epidural during childbirth. It is

---

Characteristics of hormonally triggered migraine

- Many women with hormone related attacks noticed an onset of their migraine either at puberty or in their early twenties.
- Migraines associated with the menstrual period tend to occur at the same time each month, be it mid-cycle with ovulation or at the beginning, middle or end of the period.
- Hormonally triggered migraines are often worse in the first three months of pregnancy, but thankfully (although not always) tend to ease off thereafter. (Since the safety of most medications and herbal therapies during pregnancy and while breastfeeding is not known, it is particularly important for women to consider non-drug strategies for controlling attacks during this time.)
- While going through menopause (before the periods actually stop), many women notice an increase in attacks. For many, but not all, migraines will ease off after they are completely through menopause.
- Medications that contain hormones (such as the birth-control pill, hormone-replacement therapy or medications used to treat endometriosis) affect each woman differently. They may worsen migraine, bring migraine on for the first time, not affect migraine at all or be effective in treating migraine. Their use must be carefully evaluated on an individual basis. If the attacks worsen while you are on any of these therapies, report this to your doctor without delay.

important to know that women with or without a history of migraine can suffer post-epidural headache. Migraine sufferers can experience a migraine attack after childbirth whether an epidural was used or not. Although further studies are required before any firm conclusion is reached, early reports do not show a strong increase in either post-delivery or migraine headaches in women who undergo epidural anaesthesia for childbirth.

While breastfeeding, women must continue to monitor their use of medications. Although the use of medications is not usually as limited as during pregnancy, special considerations still apply. Many doctors will authorize breastfeeding women to continue to use medications that were considered safe for use during their pregnancy. Breastfeeding women might also be able to take those medications which are commonly given directly to babies. Some doctors will prescribe preventive medicines, when necessary, to nursing mothers. In any case, it is essential to consult the doctor before taking any medications while pregnant or while breastfeeding.

Conclusions

Hormones do not *cause* migraine. A woman must already have the disorder of migraine for fluctuations in female hormones to ever trigger a migraine attack. Triggers are very individualized and not all women will find that hormonal fluctuations act as a trigger for them.

When a woman is ill, it affects her family life, her social life and her career. It is particularly important for migraine sufferers to recognize and treat migraine with the wide variety of available drug and non-drug treatments. It is important for women to take an active role in their care while working with their physicians. Women must begin by identifying and controlling exposure to known triggers, adopting regular schedules for sleeping and meal times, exercising regularly and limiting the intake of pain relievers.

5
Migraine in Infants and Children

Cathy Smith's son arrived into this world at a strapping nine and a half pounds (four kilos). He was a cheerful baby who settled into life comfortably. Outside of the usual discomforts of immunization, teething and the odd cold, he was healthy and happy.

Like many children – especially boys – Smith Jr didn't achieve night-time dryness by the time nursery school started. But the situation continued and as the years passed it became clear that bedwetting was a problem. Furthermore, Cathy was surprised on several occasions by the little figure of her son drifting through the house in episodes of sleepwalking. Sometimes he'd get sick on car trips, too. Little did Cathy know at the time that these events could be related to developing paediatric migraine.

It wasn't until about year two that he began to exhibit more concrete signs of migraine. Cathy could tell by the way he'd get off the bus that something was wrong. He'd walk up to her with his little pale face and announce that he wanted to go to bed. As they'd walk toward the house, he'd complain about his head hurting, 'and my tummy, too', and would moan about the light from the setting sun. Then he'd pack himself off to bed as soon as they got home (as Cathy wondered to herself, 'Can this be my child, who normally never stops all day long?') and would reappear feeling much better in an hour or two.

After three or four episodes of this, it was off to the doctor. Diagnosis – migraine.

It is news to many people that children, and even babies, can get migraine. Although studies vary, it is believed that 5–10 per cent of children will suffer from a migraine attack. In one famous study, a Scandinavian paediatrician found that 4 per cent of children get migraine, but an additional 6–7 per cent of the children studied suffered from frequent 'non-migrainous' headache. These percentages translate into millions of children and huge amounts of time missed from school. As well, about one-quarter of adult migraine sufferers experienced their first attack as children.

The main challenge in the care of migraine in children is arriving at the diagnosis. Since migraine is diagnosed on what the patient (and, in this case, the patient's parent or guardian) tells the doctor and, since children aren't always skilled at articulating their symptoms, many families experience difficulty obtaining the initial medical diagnosis. In addition, not all physicians are versed in the recognition of childhood migraine. But if you or a family member gets migraine, tuck away in the back of your mind the fact that migraine runs in families. Children can get migraine, and you may want to watch for symptoms, remembering that these can be distinctly different from those of adult migraine.

In childhood, more boys get migraine than girls. If you

are the parent of a child with migraine, there is reason for optimism, in that slightly less than one-third of children will stop having migraine at puberty without any action being taken. Even if it does continue (which it may, as a long-term study showed that of 73 children followed over 40 years, more than half still experienced migraine attacks at age 50), the symptoms can be controlled and the frequency of attacks reduced.

Symptoms

Children can experience the two most common forms of migraine – migraine with aura and migraine without aura. Although migraine without aura is more common, one source reports that 41 per cent of children with migraine experienced a visual warning sign. See Chapter 2 for more on auras. Children tend to experience their attacks more often than adults, some having attacks weekly or more often. Fortunately, the attacks tend to be shorter (at least four studies show a duration of only 30 minutes) but they may come on quite quickly. Many parents first notice migraine in their children when they come home from school pale and withdrawn from an attack. They may even come to suspect these attacks are triggered by active play in the schoolyard or on the way home, and often when children miss lunch or an afternoon snack.

Children's migraine pain is more likely to occur on both sides of the head, rather than on one side as often reported by adults. Often this pain is located all over the forehead or around both temples. And although adult migraine is diagnosed when there's both sensitivity to light and sensitivity to sound, children often experience one or the other –

especially younger children. The type of pain experienced by children may also be hard to assess, as qualities such as 'pulsating' are hard for children to describe. When asked to point to the location of the pain, children will often point to the entire head rather than any one particular spot.

Some authors have described a type of migraine in children called 'abdominal migraine'. This diagnosis is not accepted by most experts. Although some children experience more marked vomiting with their migraine than adults might, the notion that abdominal pain alone can be caused by migraine processes is not generally accepted. Most paediatricians agree that the most common cause of benign abdominal pain in children is constipation. All children who experience severe or recurring abdominal pain require a thorough medical examination. Migraine should not be routinely thought of as a possible primary cause.

There are rare types of childhood migraine that are recognized by the International Headache Society. These include 'alternating hemiplegia of childhood', which involves attacks of one-sided weakness on each side alternately, as well as mental impairment. Confusional migraine – a type of migraine with an aura that originates in the part of the brain that controls consciousness – may be seen as a temporary bout of inattention, distractability and difficulty maintaining speech and some motor activities. It may occur before or after the headache itself. Many of the rarer and more complicated forms of migraine described in Chapter 2 are also more common in children. Basilar migraine, for example, is mostly seen in young adults. Symptoms can include slurred speech, a decreased level of consciousness and an unsteady gait. Without knowing the medical history, a schoolteacher or emergency room physician may interpret the behaviour associated with basilar migraine to be a result of a drug or alcohol problem. Sufferers of basilar migraine should always wear a warning such as a medical-alert bracelet or tag explaining the presence of this disorder.

New children's treatment

No one, whether parent or professional, wants to give medication to a child unless it is absolutely necessary. For this reason, the treatment of most forms of migraine in children will begin with non-drug strategies – which are often highly effective in kids.

After obtaining proper medical diagnosis, the next step in dealing with children's migraine involves isolating triggers and precipitating factors. As grandmother said, 'An ounce of prevention is worth a pound of cure.'

Prevention

If it is age-appropriate, having the child keep his or her own migraine diary is very useful. Tracking attacks, times of attacks and suspected triggers may reveal a pattern over time. Consideration should be given to the possibility that a combination of triggers – rather than a single isolated one – could be to blame.

When considering the culprits that may be involved in setting off attacks, some seemingly very 'adult' causes must not be discounted. For example, many people underestimate the role that stress may play in undermining the health of children. Parents may exclaim, 'But what stress could a child possibly have?' The truth is that children do endure stress. Although the sources of childhood stress may be different, the impact is no less severe. For example, the pressures of school can seem overwhelming, particularly if the child is under great academic pressure or peer pressure, or is being bullied. Stress within the family needs to be looked at. Parents need to be careful not to advance their own agendas, which may be too demanding for the child. For instance, too many extracurricular activities may simply be too much for the child to handle in addition to a full day at school! Working with the child to develop a reasonable weekly schedule will increase the child's sense of control, and will enlist the child as an active participant in reducing headaches.

Although it is a difficult subject to discuss, physical and sexual abuse has been implicated in some cases of persistent headache disorders in children.

Establishing regular routines will go a long way to helping children with migraine. Triggers can include irregular sleep patterns, missed or delayed meals and being overtired (especially in late afternoon). Strategies to normalize the child's schedule and to allow for a good balance of activity and rest can help. Learning to relax – be it with soft music or by unwinding on the sofa with a book after supper – will prove to be a valuable skill throughout life for these – and all – children.

Although some food items have been investigated for their potential to set an attack in motion, it is widely agreed that lack of food may be the biggest food-related trigger for children. Skipping breakfast must be avoided. So must skipping lunch, a common problem in the early years when chatting is far more interesting than what is in the lunch box. Keeping pace with caloric requirements for sports and the rapid growth of adolescence is crucial. If there aren't enough calories going in regularly, migraine sufferers will easily fall victim to frequent attacks.

When a severe attack strikes, parents often feel at a loss as to what to do. Wendy Gage, of the neurology clinic at the Hospital for Sick Children in Toronto, Canada, offers parents and kids assistance to identify and change their beliefs about pain. She helps children learn to perceive the experience of pain in a way that reduces their fear and anxiety and leads to more control over both the situation and the pain itself.

Through Wendy's experience with hundreds of children and families with migraine, she has developed a practical list of 'dos and don'ts' for parents whose children are in the throes of a migraine:

Do . . .

- believe the child who complains of a headache. It is very frightening when the parent doesn't reinforce a child's reality. Faking is rare and, if it is present, children will only 'up the ante' if parents question whether the pain is real. Restating the symptoms – 'Oh, you aren't well', or 'My, you have a headache' – is comforting.

- calm the child. Holding, touching and massage can help. It is important for the parents to control their own emotions, too – the child will pick up on the parents' panic and become frightened by the parents' discomfort.

- give the child choices, especially where treatment is concerned. Although it is tempting to take over, allowing the child to be in control is important. For example, you could offer treatment choice: 'Would you rather lie down on the couch or in your bed? Would you like an icepack? Do you want some medication?' Older children and adolescents need more space and it is important for the parent to back off to foster the development of independent management strategies. This is the 'I'm here when you need me' approach.

- help the child break down the task of eliminating the headache by focusing on pain reduction first, before pain elimination is attempted. Wendy's analogy is 'You can't eat an elephant whole – but if you ate it bite by bite, eventually you would eat the whole elephant.' Ask the child to focus on reducing the headache a bit for a specified period of time – say an hour. Provide positive reinforcement as he or she uses pain reduction strategies, and encourage the child to go on to the next stage to reduce the pain even more. When this technique works, it works well. However, sometimes the attack is just too stubborn, and the child should be encouraged and praised for these efforts nonetheless.

- talk about the pain and show understanding of it. Provide reassurance that the pain is real and that it is *not* life-threatening. Wendy has treated children whose primary belief was that their pain came from a brain tumour, even when imaging had been done and a tumour had been ruled out.

- consider learning relaxation and imagery techniques. These can be very effective pain management strategies, especially in children.

Don't . . .

- mollycoddle. Don't fall over yourself to do for the child what he or she can reasonably do unassisted. Tasks such as making the bed or carrying dishes to the sink will show the child that life hasn't ground to a halt.

- provide 'secondary gain'. If the child is home sick, the child is home sick. Presents, treats and trips should not result from a migraine. Interestingly, the children that Wendy treats have told her that they are frightened when parents start allowing treats and behaviours normally not allowed. For instance, one young girl thought things must be *really bad* when Mum allowed Sugar-puffs! Normalizing life as much as possible during the pain is important, to prevent kids from either capitalizing on time off school, or being frightened that something worse is happening to them than they are being told. Children have very vivid imaginations!

• take away children's control over themselves and their environment.

The role of medications

If these techniques do not bring relief, doctors and parents may consider treating childhood migraine with medication. Medication is usually considered only if the child's play or school work is disrupted. Doctors may prescribe medication such as paracetamol or ibuprofen, which has been shown to be superior for pain or domperidone for vomiting, in some cases. Prescription pain relievers or anti-nausea preparations are occasionally given (beware of the rebound effect in children as well – see Chapter 2). Preventive medications may be considered if the migraine is significantly and regularly affecting the child's ability to carry on his or her daily life (see Chapter 8).

Dr Daune MacGregor, a paediatric neurologist at the Hospital for Sick Children, Toronto, recommends that many of her patients take simple analgesics such as paracetamol or ibuprofen at the onset of the headache, in appropriate doses. But she cautions the children (and/or the parents, if they are to administer the medication) not to dose the headache repeatedly. For instance, if ibuprofen is given and there isn't good relief, she recommends trying paracetamol in four hours' time. Dr MacGregor recommends that no more than two doses of the same or different medication be given in any four to six hours. This entire regimen should not be administered more than twice a week. If the headaches occur more often than this and all efforts are being made to avoid triggers and precipitating factors to no avail, it could be that prescription medications are warranted.

Once an attack is in progress, narcotics such as codeine or pethidine are generally counterproductive in children's migraine, as they can lead to chronic persistent headache disorders and/or mask other illnesses. The triptan group of medications is sometimes used in children, although these drugs don't have formal regulatory approval for paediatric use. There is some recent evidence that nasal sumatriptan may be helpful for adolescent migraine.

More commonly, preventive medications – although they too have not been thoroughly studied or formally approved – are considered when a prescription is necessary. Preventives such as cyproheptadine, propranolol, pizotyline or pizotifen, valproic acid and gabapentin may be considered (see Chapter 8 for descriptions). Some doctors are trying riboflavin prophylaxis, as described in Chapter 10, with adjusted doses for children, and it is theoretically possible that children may one day be helped by botulinum toxin injections (Chapter 8).

As a parent of a migraine sufferer, you will want to 'be there' for your child. You will attempt to make him or her comfortable and explain the disorder to family and teachers. Consult your doctor about the diagnosis of migraine in your child. Your doctor may be able to pinpoint overlooked triggers or recommend medication to help during an attack, or to prevent or reduce the number of attacks. Remember that your family is not alone.

Children and their parents' migraine

A 1998 study by Dr R. Smith examined the impact of migraine on the family. One of the groups studied included families with children under the age of 12. The results were revealing: when migraine struck a parent, one-quarter of the children felt confused, 17 per cent were hostile and 12 per cent felt afraid. In many cases (61 per cent), the affected parent was unable to care for the children at all.

For small children, the thought of either mother or father leaving can be frightening. Children rely on their parents for physical, emotional and spiritual assistance and guidance on a daily basis. It stands to reason that they can become quite fearful when their mother or father falls ill.

Many of us underestimate the capacity of a child's mind. Adults are often shocked about what comes 'out of the mouths of babes', as a child's interpretation of a situation or event is often unobscured by pretence and can be quite blunt. Children also have vivid imaginations and may harbour fearful thoughts that parents wouldn't even imagine. For instance, if a grandparent or parent has to go to the hospital for minor surgery or a test, a child may think the worst and be afraid that the person will never come home again.

Children may become fearful about who will take care of them when a parent is sick. Some children come to believe that they are somehow to blame for a parent's illness. Although these thoughts may seem irrational to an adult, they can seem very real to a child.

Children whose parents are ill require explanation of what is happening. They need to know that Mummy's or Daddy's headache will pass and that she or he will be fine in no time. The child should know that it's 'just one of those things' and not anyone's fault. The child must be told who will be temporarily taking over the parent's duties. It may be possible to present the change in routine as being 'fun' – for instance, having lunch at Grandma's house when Mummy is sick could be presented as a special event.

If the child is at home when the parent is ill, consider assigning a simple task so that he or she can feel helpful (I remember bringing my bedridden mother a sliced orange during one of her migraine attacks). Being allowed to see that the parent is resting in bed (and looking okay) is reassuring. Once the child is satisfied, he or she can be encouraged to play quietly to keep the noise level down.

Importantly, the impact of migraine on the whole family – and not just the person directly affected – needs to be considered.

6
Getting Older, Getting Better

Migraine sufferers tend to feel *better* as they get older! The reason for this good news isn't completely understood, but it is believed to be a result of normal chemical changes within the brain, which accompany ageing. For women, menopause can eliminate the hormonal fluctuations that may have been triggering attacks, leaving the sufferer virtually headache free. For some women, however, the attacks can worsen while they are going through 'the change', and, for a few, migraine can actually begin at menopause.

Those who get migraine with aura may find that, as they age, they continue to have the aura but not the headache that used to follow. This type of 'migraine without headache' can also occur for the first time in people who have never had migraine, although it is usually investigated in the older population to rule out the possibility of the symptoms being caused by 'mini-strokes' (known medically as 'transient ischaemic attacks', or TIAs). Usually the visual signs of aura develop gradually if the cause is migraine and more suddenly if caused by TIAs. (Migraine and TIAs are not related.)

Migraine typically begins in adolescence. Rarely, however, it can start later in life. As a general rule of thumb, doctors tend to investigate more thoroughly headaches that begin after the age of 50 to rule out other causes of head pain. If the diagnosis is migraine, the treatment plan for the older sufferer is the same as for a younger migraineur, except for some extra limitations on the medications used.

Since a narrowing of the arteries normally occurs in us all at different rates as we age, some of the medications that further constrict blood vessels to treat migraine are avoided in the older population. Ergotamines, for instance, are not usually prescribed much past the age of 55. The manufacturer's guidelines advise that sumatriptan is not recommended for people over age 65. Of course, doctors may recommend the use of some of these medications in older patients if the benefits outweigh the risks, and if there is no history or high risk of heart disease or stroke present.

When considering migraine medication of any type, it is important that your doctor knows about all your other health problems. Many medications used for the treatment of migraine should not be used in the presence of other health problems. For instance, beta-adrenergic blockers should not be used by asthmatics. Many people feel silly having their chest listened to or their abdomen examined when they go to the doctor to see about their headache. But the doctor may want to examine other areas to get a picture of a patient's overall health status.

It is also important for the doctor and chemist to know about all the medications being taken (including non-prescription preparations) in order to avoid negative drug interactions. Of course, when getting a new prescription, it's always good to remind the doctor and chemist of any allergies you have.

The risk of new headache being caused by disorders other than benign headaches (such as migraine or tension-type headache) increases as we age. For this reason, it is even more important for older people to see the doctor right away about any new symptoms or a change in existing symptoms if they already suffer from a headache disorder. Although older people can experience migraine or any of the other types of benign headache disorders mentioned in this book, other causes of head or face pain in the elderly may include the following:

- *Arthritis of the jaw or neck* can cause moderate to severe pain. Arthritic pain does not throb. Arthritic pain can 'flare up' from time to time, and may be worse in damp weather.
- *Chronic lung problems* such as emphysema can cause headaches if the person's oxygen levels are low.
- *Dental problems* such as tooth decay, abscess, deterioration of the joint in the jaw or problems with chewing can cause pain. Additionally, 'phantom' tooth pain, or pain in a tooth that is no longer there (and may have been lost many years ago), can cause pain through mechanisms that are not fully understood.
- *Fever of any origin*, whether caused by a virus or bacteria invading any part of the body, can cause a headache.
- *Neuralgia* is pain that travels along the course of a nerve. Neuralgia can cause intense stabbing pain in the face as well as in other areas of the body. Usually the pain is so severe that the person seeks medical attention without delay.
- *Side effects of some medications* can include headache. Check with the doctor or chemist.
- *Sinus infections* can cause head pain, face pain, pain around the eyes, fever and a runny and/or stuffy nose.

Sinus infections are not usually the cause of headaches that come and go for years (many people who think they suffer from intermittent sinus headache are actually migraine sufferers – true sinus headache is always accompanied by an infection that can be detected by the doctor).

- *Strokes, brain tumours, brain aneurysms (ballooning of a blood vessel) and other life-threatening problems* can also cause headaches. Fortunately, they are rarely found to be at the root of headaches.
- *Temporal arteritis* (inflammation of an artery) is a medical condition found almost exclusively among the older population. A doctor can diagnose this condition, which is associated with a headache. A specific blood test will be done as part of the diagnostic check-up.
- *Viral infections*, including colds and the flu, can cause headache. The fever often accompanying such infection may cause headache on its own or in combination with the actual virus.

This list of potential causes of headache other than migraine or other benign types of headache in the older population is intended as a call to action if new head pain arises. Remember, the earlier you seek medical attention, the better the outcome is likely to be.

7
Steps in Self-Management

The very first step in conquering migraine involves making a firm commitment to take control of your situation. This means being the number-one person in charge of all aspects of migraine treatment and prevention. It also means taking the responsibility for finding all the available expertise, help and talent of healthcare providers. Once the best team possible is assembled, you must actively participate in decisions made regarding your own care. You must ultimately become the ongoing manager of your own migraine treatment plan. To become a self-manager, you must become an informed participant. Self-education is a key component of health for migraine sufferers.

Migraine education

Few fears are worse than the one shared by most sufferers of recurring headache – namely, being diagnosed as having a brain tumour. The mere thought of cancer invading one's brain, undergoing brain surgery and facing one's mortality is enough to overshadow the rational knowledge that less than 2 per cent of all headaches are caused by underlying lesions. Someone who has not received reassurance through proper diagnosis of benign headache, or who is not well educated about migraine, may live in fear of the cause of the pain. Even migraine sufferers who know that they've got another migraine may still hear the voice of doubt from time to time saying, 'Maybe I've developed a brain tumour.' It is important to realize and to remember that migraine has a *primary* origin – that is, it is not caused by something else, such as a growth. Migraine is, in itself, a neurochemical disorder.

A study by Dr Russell Packard, published in a 1979 edition of *Headache*, the journal of the American Association for the Study of Headache, asked 50 doctors why they thought their headache patients came to see them. Fifty-six per cent of the doctors surveyed said their patients wanted pain relief. Twenty-two per cent of the doctors said their patients wanted an explanation for their headache pain. When a hundred headache patients were asked why they had sought a doctor's advice, 46 per cent said they wanted an explanation and only 31 per cent actually expected pain relief. This study underscores the universal need for information about the pain of migraine. Satisfying this need is one of the most important steps in migraine management.

Migraine sufferers have been frustrated by the lack of adequate information about, and explanation of, migraine and its treatment. Fortunately, the medical community has become much more committed to headache education since the 1970s, but headache patients must learn about their disorder and take responsibility for informing family members and close friends about the impact migraine has on their lives. There is far more information available than could possibly be absorbed during a typical doctor's appointment or while standing at the chemist's counter. The patient who takes an active role in studying migraine constantly discovers more about the disorder and stands a much better chance of gaining control over his or her particular symptoms. Sources of information on migraine may include handouts at the doctor's office, leaflets enclosed with certain migraine medications and, of course, books like this one or others available in stores or at libraries. One of the most helpful pieces of advice that can be given to a migraine sufferer is to read, read, read. Family members, friends, colleagues and employers who want to 'do something' for the migraine sufferer in their lives could broaden their understanding by reading on the subject. Even if you've encountered the information before, the reassurance of seeing it in black and white or seeing it restated in different ways by different authors helps to quiet that doubting voice in the back of the mind that says, 'What if . . . ?' during a bad attack. Reassurance gives migraine sufferers the strength of knowing they are not alone in suffering from this medical disorder. Also, by keeping up to date, you can avail yourself of the growing body of knowledge emerging through medical research.

Do not limit yourself to reading literature and books specifically about migraine. By researching and discovering information on medicines, complementary therapies, the management of persistent pain disorders or other related topics, many migraine sufferers pick up practical tips. And in the spirit of 'It takes one to know one,' sharing information with other sufferers is vital, be it informally with a family member, friend or acquaintance with migraine, through participation in a self-help group or through publications.

Migraine and guilt

Even when diagnosed properly, many migraine sufferers feel that they have somehow given themselves the disorder. They blame themselves when an attack strikes and interferes with plans. Some fear making plans because they will feel guilty if they are forced to cancel. Some worry so much that they simply cannot look forward to any planned events. The self-blame involved with many people's migraine often leads to feelings of guilt. Ensuing feelings of helplessness, anxiety and depression are all too often reported. Some sufferers even believe that migraine is a punishment for past sins, or that they deserve to feel ill as they have not been the 'good person' they thought they should be.

The guilt felt by many migraine sufferers is likely a result of self-esteem being undermined by society's lack of acceptance of migraine as the *bona fide* medical disorder that it is. But there is a way to help end the guilt. It is important for all migraine sufferers to educate themselves, to re-educate themselves and to stay current in their knowledge of the true causes of migraine – causes that are not, by any means, self-induced. Migraine sufferers must remind themselves *and* teach those around them that migraine is a neurobiochemical disorder caused by a largely inborn - chemical disruption. They must learn the most effective ways to avoid and overcome as much as possible their particular patterns of migraine attacks, and not to blame themselves for the attacks that occur despite their very best efforts.

It has been said: 'Guilt is a wasted, self-induced emotion.'

Migraine and fear

Various fears plague migraine sufferers from time to time. The fear of having a life-threatening problem such as a tumour or aneurysm crosses the minds of even the most long-standing migraine sufferers during their weaker moments. Remember, potentially life-threatening causes of head pain are rare.

Something that lurks at the very root of migraine is fear of the next attack. Migraine strikes without warning and those prone to it can never be sure when the next attack will come. When migraine arrives, they can never be sure how severe the symptoms will be. In its most severe forms, migraine can be frightfully painful. Sufferers of migraine with aura may find the symptoms of the aura to be disturbing. Those who experience the more dramatic types of migraine, such as basilar or hemiplegic migraine, may find themselves frightened by their symptoms.

The secret to keeping these fears at bay lies in a proper diagnosis and a thorough understanding of the processes of migraine through adequate education. With the reassurance of a firm diagnosis and the intellectual knowledge that migraine is a benign disorder, sufferers are armed to do battle with their darkest fears. In addition, by making efforts towards understanding symptoms and reducing the frequency and severity of attacks, migraine sufferers can also reduce their fears about when the next attack will hit.

The triggers of migraine

Medical research has proven that migraine is a biological disorder of the brain. Individuals with migraine have an inborn proneness to recurring painful attacks of head pain and the other symptoms of migraine. People with low prone-ness will have infrequent attacks. Headache proneness can be reduced to a certain extent, but the key to reducing the number of attacks lies in the identification and elimination (where possible) of migraine triggers – factors that are capable of starting a migraine attack.

We know that the mechanism of migraine involves a complex relationship between nerve impulses, chemical transmitters (predominantly serotonin) and blood vessels. The mechanism of migraine can begin to fire for reasons that are not apparent or it can be kicked off in response to migraine triggers. There are two main types of triggers: trig-gers external to the sufferer (such as the chemical content of certain foods, bright lights or weather patterns) and internal triggers (such as female hormones, changes in sleep patterns or the body's response to stress). These triggers are interpreted by the body and brain as either real or potential threats of tissue injury.

Triggers are very individual and, although there is a common thread, what sparks an attack for some may have no effect on others. For instance, some women will have a worsening of their migraine around the time of the men-strual period; others won't. Some people court disaster by eating chocolate, where others can happily munch away without ill consequences. Migraine sufferers must become 'trigger detectives' to identify exactly what factors influence their individual headache proneness.

The trigger investigation

What is triggering migraine attacks is usually not obvious. In an attempt to discover the culprits, some have kept long lists of everything they ate, drank, did, saw and felt, and what happened to them daily for some months. Meticulous record-keeping such as this doesn't usually pay off, simply because there is too much information to sift through (a case of not being able to see the wood for the trees). Others have taken the 'elimination' route, particularly where diet is concerned. Diets that advocate reducing intake to the least potentially reactive foods, such as rice, pears, and bottled water, then reintroducing foods slowly while monitoring reactions, tend to be extreme. They also don't take into consideration that we can't isolate ourselves during the experiment, and that other factors may be at work on the migraine at the same time (such as hormonal fluctuations or weather-pattern changes). Most experts today agree that the most sensible and practical approach for identifying triggers involves examining for several attacks the 24 to 48 hours preceding each attack.

Other important information to record may include any medications or treatments used during the attack, and the responses experienced. After this information has been kept for several attacks, patterns of triggers can sometimes be discerned. One mother of a young rugby player discovered that her attacks occurred most often on Saturdays. She attributed the start of the attack to the weekend commotion surrounding getting her son to practice, the noise and shouts during practice, delaying and sometimes skipping meals – resulting in grabbing a sausage or other on-the-run food – often loaded with preservatives. Although some of the triggers remained unavoidable in the face of healthy young boys' enthusiasm, she reduced her attacks by taking her usual meals when possible and by avoiding additive-rich snacks. Wearing sunglasses on the field also helped reduce glare. Frequently, it is the cumulative effect of different triggers rather than any single one that brings on an attack. The principle of 'the straw that broke the camel's back' explains why you may get away with a chocolate bar on one day, but fall victim to a roaring attack if it's washed down with a glass of wine after a disrupted night's sleep.

Many migraine sufferers instinctively know when it's a 'bad day'. On these days, they sense that they must be careful to keep that 'twinge' of a headache just below the surface from erupting. You may be able to stave off attacks by eliminating any known and avoidable triggers on 'bad days'.

Clues for trigger detectives

In this section, we examine the most commonly reported migraine triggers. Not all will apply, and the listing is purposely somewhat exhaustive. Even so, you may find that

---

Migraine detective work

When a migraine strikes, sufferers are advised to start their detective work by writing down the following information concerning the preceding two days:

- food consumed (including snacks)
- beverages consumed
- missed meals
- activities
- changes to normal routine (such as travel)
- any particular surprises, excitement or stressors
- time spent relaxing
- sleep patterns
- day of the week
- for women, days since the start of the last menstrual period
- exposure to bright sunlight or loud noise
- weather patterns, particularly storms or approaching storms
- any other factors the individual may suspect to be triggers.

your triggers are not mentioned, as triggers can be as individual as snowflakes. Migraine sufferers must continue to monitor their response to triggers throughout life. As the body changes with age, triggers may also change.

Dietary

Perhaps the most traditional triggers to which attention has been paid are the potential dietary ones. Although actual scientific evidence of the ability of substances to act as triggers is scarce, the chemical content of certain foods seems to play a role. Nevertheless, one source states that food is a factor in less than 10 per cent of migraine attacks.

Many people confuse food's role in migraine with allergy. Frequently sufferers say, 'I'm allergic to that food; it will give me a migraine.' As we have seen, migraine and allergy are not related. A food allergy results in allergic responses – hives, watery eyes, wheezing, etc. When food acts as a migraine trigger, it is frequently the chemical content of the food or a reaction in the body that acts to kick off the migraine response.

Frequently, the chemical in food that causes migraine-sensitive blood vessels to react is tyramine. Many migraine sufferers choose to stick to a diet that is as tyramine-free as possible. Tyramine is a vasoactive substance – that is, it can dilate blood vessels. Sources of tyramine include pods of broad beans, pickled herring, chicken liver, mature cheese, alcoholic beverages, bananas, raisins, figs, yeasts, consommé and bouillon, soy sauce, yoghurt and sour cream. Citrus fruits contain a vasoactive substance called 'octopamine'. Another culprit is histamine. Histamine sources include wine, beer, fish, certain cheeses, cured sausage and pickled cabbage. Preservatives such as monosodium glutamate (MSG, found in many commercially prepared foods and soups) and nitrites (found in cured meats) can spell trouble.

Remember that food does not cause migraine; rather, migraine is caused by the inborn proneness to attacks. But certain foods may act as a trigger. Some of the more common culprits include:

- mature cheese
- red wine and other coloured alcohols (contain histamine and by-products which form in the drinks as they are aged)
- chocolate (contains tyramine and another vasoactive substance, phenylethylamine)
- food additives (possibly because of their chemical effects on blood vessels) such as nitrites, found in preserved meats and hot dogs, and MSG, found in many canned, packaged and fast foods, and as a component of soy sauce; read labels carefully
- other foods such as certain vegetables (notably onions, tomatoes and beans), nuts, citrus fruits (oranges, lemons, grapefruit), homemade breads and the artificial sweetener aspartame, also cited as common triggers, although evidence is once again not conclusively proven or explained
- caffeine-containing beverages (caffeine increases the body's sensitivity to painful stimuli)
- sudden withdrawal from caffeine-containing beverages (this is known as the rebound effect; it is thought that caffeine-withdrawal rebound headaches result after regular consumption is stopped in those who regularly drink six or more cups of coffee per day – or an equivalent intake of 480 milligrams or more of caffeine per day).

The apparent dilemma of both caffeine and caffeine-withdrawal acting as triggers may be eliminated by tapering off caffeine consumption, reducing pain sensitivity but avoiding rebound from the sudden withdrawal of caffeine. The small amounts of caffeine added to some painkillers or the cup of strong coffee used for medicinal reasons at the beginning of an attack does not usually have harmful effects.

Those who seek to avoid caffeine-related difficulty in sleeping should not expect a full reprieve from switching to decaffeinated coffee. Coffee contains other chemicals that may have stimulating effects.

Some people have suggested replacing migraine-triggering foods with ones less likely to cause problems rather than depriving oneself entirely. For example, although it is the subject of debate, some claim that carob makes a non-triggering substitute for chocolate. Probably the most practical advice is for sufferers to monitor themselves for individual reactions to foods, or to substitute other foods for suspected triggers.

Fasting or skipping or delaying meals can cause a drop in blood sugar, which can kick off an attack. The fall in the blood-sugar level may be so slight that it doesn't show up

Caffeine levels – obvious and not

Migraine sufferers should be aware of the hidden levels of caffeine in some products. The following listing of caffeine levels may prove helpful:

Coffee (6 oz/180 ml)	80–175 mg
Instant coffee (6 oz/180 ml)	60–100 mg
Decaffeinated coffee (6 oz/180 ml)	2–5 mg
Tea (6 oz/180 ml)	20–100 mg
Hot chocolate (6 oz/180 ml)	2–20 mg
Cola (12 oz/355 ml)	30–45 mg
Milk chocolate (1 oz/28 g)	1–10 mg
Dark chocolate (1 oz/28 g)	5–35 mg
Chocolate cake, per serving (6 oz/170 g)	20–30 mg

on routine tests for hypoglycaemia; nevertheless, the drop could be enough to act as a trigger. To help keep blood-sugar levels stable, eat small meals about four hours apart during the day, including late in the evening, before bedtime, rather than having three larger meals a day (the quantity of food consumed will be the same). Eating fresh vegetables, fibrous fruit, whole grains and proteins may help to stabilize sugar levels. Avoid refined sugars as much as possible. As well, crash dieting and fad diets are out of the question for those affected by low blood sugar. In any case, a programme of gradual weight loss aimed at reducing the intake of fat and increasing the intake of fibre is a more sensible strategy for all dieters.

Changes

The body of a migraine sufferer is particularly sensitive to change, and alterations in schedule can kick off a migraine attack for some people. An area within the brain known as the hypothalamus functions as the body's own clock. Despite what the hands on the wall clock say, your body follows its own time. The body knows when you should be sleeping, and will react if it doesn't get treated with regularity. Migraine sufferers will, on average, feel better simply by setting and adhering to a regular schedule for sleeping, rising and eating meals. It is best not to deviate more than an hour each way for any of these events. For most, this will mean forgoing sleeping in on weekends. As with everything else, there will be times when you simply can't stick to a regimented schedule (or don't want to – for example, when a late night out may be worth the gamble of triggering a migraine). Shift workers may not be able to regulate their hours of sleep. But, by and large, efforts made towards the goal of keeping a regular schedule for sleeping, waking and eating are likely to pay off.

Travel, particularly air travel across time zones, often presents a challenge. It has been said that it takes one day to adjust for each hour lost or gained travelling across time zones (so if there's a four-hour time difference, travellers should give themselves four days before they can expect to feel 'in sync'). Frequent flyers have suggested the following tips to help avoid migraine on airplanes:

- drink plenty of water while in the air
- bring your own food to avoid any food additives
- if it's not possible to bring your own food, request a cold salad plate
- don't drink alcohol
- get up and move around as frequently as possible
- book a non-smoking flight.

When away on holiday, take along enough medication and any equipment required for non-drug therapies you are currently using. As well, try to adhere to a meal and sleep schedule as much as possible.

If there is room in the suitcase, consider bringing along your own pillow. This added comfort may prevent rock-hard or pancake-flat hotel pillows from triggering neck problems that may lead to a migraine attack.

Emotional triggers

Probably the hardest myth to dispel is the belief that migraine is *caused* by stress. Although migraine is certainly not caused by stress, evidence is growing that stress has a negative impact on our bodies and health. Just as stress can worsen the health of a person with asthma or cancer, stress can worsen migraine. The body's reaction to stress and to the release of stress can act to set a migraine into motion. Migraine sufferers are advised to be diligent in their efforts to change any 'Type A' behaviours (perfectionistic, driven, 'life in the fast lane' or overly serious behaviours), and to make sincere attempts at taking a more relaxed approach to living. Behavioural modification techniques can prove helpful: learning better time-management strategies at home and at the office, increasing time spent with family and friends, taking up hobbies and pursuing pleasurable activities. Counsellors can also help people to take a positive approach and attitude to handling the stresses of day-to-day life. Persistent pain such as migraine may respond to relaxation and biofeedback techniques, which can help to prevent attacks and can also help in coping with pain when it does occur. If stress is a trigger, adequate rest *and* regular exercise become vital weapons. It is also important to stay away from stimulants such as caffeine and to limit intake of refined sugars.

It is not clear whether the release of adrenaline during stress is what triggers an attack. This doubt comes largely from the phenomenon known as the 'come-down-from-stress' migraine. Many people go through a period of excitement or stress without an attack, but fall victim to a migraine after the event is over. Many migraine sufferers have an attack on the first day or so of a holiday, or after a particularly stressful work week. (The culprit in weekend migraine may be the come-down effect alone, or coupled with the negative effects of changes to the usual sleep pattern from oversleeping and/or a withdrawal from caffeine when the usual early-morning jolt of tea or coffee is delayed.) We don't know why a come-down from stress induces migraine, but it has become accepted that it can be a trigger. The solution? Try to avoid the peaks and valleys when possible, practical and desirable (after all, these periods of excitement can be 'good stressors' too). Sticking to as regular a schedule as possible for going to bed and getting up in the morning, even on weekends and holidays, may also improve the way you feel.

Depression and other coexisting medical conditions

Although it is true that psychological factors should not be emphasized as the *cause* of migraine, the underlying biological root of migraine *is* related to the same biochemical processes involved with other disorders such as depression. It may be as a result of this biochemical root that some researchers point to a higher incidence of depression in migraine sufferers than in those who do not get migraine. This relationship may be even higher among those who develop chronic daily headache. It may be the defect in serotonin metabolism in both disorders that causes the relationship. One study showed that panic attacks are 12 times more likely to occur in people with a history of migraine, even if the migraine has been in remission for a year or more. Other health problems that may be chemically related to migraine (some of which may be more likely to coexist in migraine sufferers) include anxiety, sleep disorders, mood disorders, obsessive-compulsive disorders, fibromyalgia (muscle pain), chronic fatigue syndrome, vestibular Ménière's disease (an inner-ear disease that causes hearing loss and attacks of dramatic dizziness), Raynaud's phenomenon (intermittent episodes of constriction of small blood vessels of the extremities, usually the fingers – skin on extremity becomes cold and discoloured) and irritable bowel syndrome. Epilepsy is about twelve times more common among people with migraine than it is in the general population.

Good psychological health does have a role to play in migraine. Many people have difficulty seeking the help of a counsellor in working through any issues that may be involved. There is an outdated stigma attached to consulting psychiatrists and psychologists. In fact, talking over problems and feelings with a professional can help to identify the sources of difficulties, and the counsellor can help to find fresh solutions to the bigger hurdles in life.

Many migraine sufferers report that, although 'having a good cry' can be a therapeutic way of working through difficult situations, crying can sometimes lead to a headache. Although the mechanism behind this is not understood, it may be related to the come-down-from-stress phenomenon.

Hormones

Migraine affects two or three times as many women as men. The reason is believed to be the influence of female hormones on the chemical balance underlying migraine. Attempts throughout the years to 'normalize' the hormonal level through oestrogen addition or the removal of oestrogen through hysterectomy have often met with failure in treating migraine. Unacceptable side effects have often developed as well. Hormonally triggered migraine is one of the more difficult types of migraine to treat as there is no way of avoiding the release of hormones. Not all triggers of migraine are controllable. If the trigger is the hormonal fluctuations of a woman's menstrual cycle, her best defence is to minimize her exposure to triggers that are within her control (such as chocolate) to prevent the additive effect that triggers have. But if the hormonal trigger is identifiable and removable (such as the hormone increase from the birth-control pill), a decision may be made to discontinue using the pill. See Chapter 4 for more on hormonal influences on migraine in women.

Weather

Weather may have a profound influence on migraine attacks. It has been demonstrated that a particular kind of weather – weather characterized by low barometric pressure; the passage of a warm front; high temperature and humidity; and often drizzly, overcast skies – is associated with a higher number of migraine attacks and a worsening of migraine attacks that were in progress before the weather change.

The same study found that barometric pressure alone did not exert a profound influence on migraine. The research points more to the effects of weather systems than to individual weather components. But anecdotal evidence indicates that a huge number of migraine sufferers find that rapid changes in barometric pressure spell trouble. For most it's when the barometer is falling and a storm is approaching, but some say that it's when the barometer is rising and we're pulling out of the storm and headed for a very sunny day. Hot, dry winds – such as the Swedish Föhn, the Mediterranean Meltemi and the Canadian Chinook – have long been associated with headache and general irritability. Migraine sufferers often make reliable human barometers – many swear that they feel the changes in weather as much as twenty-four hours before they are detected at the weather station!

Recent research into the effects of weather on health has

led to a growing interest in the field of biometeorology – the study of the impact of weather on health. In countries such as Germany, people with particular health problems can access information on weather patterns to help them plan their day, or make any possible adjustments to their plans if the weather indicates a high trigger risk.

When the forecast is for a storm, stay away from other avoidable triggers so that you have a better chance of standing up to the effects of the weather. Staying indoors will not help in avoiding the effects of the weather, since pressure changes and other factors occur inside buildings as well.

The great outdoors

Migraine sufferers should consider taking a few simple extra precautions when outdoors. The glare of sunlight can act as a migraine trigger. A dark pair of sunglasses is usually the answer. Strong wind against the head (particularly cold wind) can set migraine into motion. Protecting yourself with a scarf or balaclava may help.

Odours

Odours that normally seem ordinary or even pleasant can become overpowering (hyperosmia) during an attack or can smell foul (osmophobia). Odour as a precipitant of migraine was first described by William Gowers in 1888. The British Migraine Association showed that 15 of its 80 members have their migraine triggered by an odour. Odours most commonly cited as triggers include perfume and paint. Another study showed that 40 per cent of migraine sufferers experience a dislike of particular odours during an attack. Exposure to that particular odour during an attack will cause the sufferer's head to throb with greater intensity.

Migraine can cause a heightened sensitivity to smells. Some sufferers find their sense of smell changes during an attack. Odours that are normally considered pleasant may become offensive during a migraine. In rare cases, a hallucination of a particular smell may occur when an attack is approaching. These smells can be very individual.

Everyday situations may become a problem. People who are sensitive to the scent of perfume must avoid the perfume counter in department stores, but many stores place the perfume section right near the ground-floor entrance! Shopping during the Christmas season can create an added strain for sufferers, as these counters are staffed with even more people offering perfume samples to passers-by. Shopping by catalogue may save a few trips out into the crowds.

Magazines often include scented strips as part of a perfume company's advertising feature. Open the pages and a heavy whiff of scent blows your way. Fortunately, subscribers to many magazines can now ask to receive scent-free issues.

You may face a difficult situation if a colleague wears a particular perfume or cologne, but you must find a delicate way to voice your concerns. First, you could compliment them on their selection. Then explain that, although the scent is quite appealing, it is acting to trigger a health problem in you. Tell them that you suffer incapacitating migraine attacks that can be set in motion by a variety of triggers. Explain that, like people with diabetes whose blood sugar goes haywire if they eat a big piece of chocolate cake, migraine sufferers can have attacks when exposed to certain odours, and that perfume is one of them. Explain that, for this reason, you are not able to wear perfume yourself. Elicit their co-operation. They will understand only if you provide them with information about migraine and your particular sensitivity to perfume. Suggest to them that they bring the perfume to work so they can put it on before going home at the end of the day.

Tobacco smoke – especially pipe and cigar smoke – can be a brutal irritant during a migraine. Fortunately, smoke-free zones are growing more common. Smoke does not cause the same problems as perfume in the workplace owing to by-laws in most areas. If you are a smoke-sensitive sufferer, you should seek a smoke-free workplace and smoke-free restaurant seating. If you live with a smoker, send him or her out to the balcony or garden to smoke. In any case, there is abundant evidence that secondhand smoke is a health risk in general.

Redecorating or moving into a new house or apartment is exciting. However, fresh paint (particularly oil-based paint) can act as a trigger. Paint must be applied only in well-ventilated areas. The scent of new carpeting is believed to cause headaches in certain people. To help prevent the scent of a new or newly redecorated home from triggering an attack, it is imperative to open the windows, and sleeping with an open window for at least the first week is a good idea. During warm weather, doing so is not difficult, and it may be possible to sleep with the window open a crack during cold weather. However, some sufferers simply have to sleep somewhere else for the first few nights after paint is applied or a new carpet is laid.

Other factors

Loud noise, bright lights and flashing lights can act as triggers. The taste of certain foods can be thrown off during an attack. Many migraine sufferers cannot tolerate the motion of carnival rides, swings or boats (most can't even imagine going anywhere near them during attacks).

Other health problems can trigger migraine attacks simply by worsening a person's overall health, thereby making him or her more prone to attacks. Structural problems in the neck or jaw, as in temporomandibular disorder (TMD), can act as triggers. (Temporomandibular disorder used to be called temporomandibular joint syndrome, or TMJ.) The treatment of TMD is usually carried out by a dentist. Although TMD does not cause migraine and less than 5 per cent of people with TMD have associated headaches, some people have reported relief from their migraine from addressing the problems in the jaw that may have been acting as a migraine trigger. Unfortunately, migraine sufferers only rarely receive relief from their migraine through correction of TMD. However, if the TMD is causing symptoms such as clicking and pain in the jaw, difficulty chewing, or facial pain or earaches, having it assessed may be in order. Treatment is required by only 5 per cent of those with TMD, and may involve wearing dental appliances such as bite plates or splints that are fitted over the teeth. If the TMD is caused by clenching or grinding of the teeth (usually during sleep), measures to gain control over stress may be suggested. Surgery may be performed as a last resort in extreme cases. Several opinions should be sought before proceeding with any type of surgery.

Attention to proper posture is important for migraineurs. Proper body alignment, particularly in the neck and upper-body areas, is important. Sufferers who sit at a desk all day or are forced to stand or perform repetitive movements during the workday must pay attention to proper body mechanics and must be sure to change their position and stretch out stressed areas during break times.

People who wake in the morning with headaches not related to caffeine withdrawal, excessive use of pain relievers or oversleeping may wish to investigate 'orthopaedic' pillows, which may help to protect the neck from strain while sleeping. Trying such commercially available pillows will involve trial and error. To date, no particular type has been proven especially helpful for migraineurs – it's a matter of personal preference.

If undergoing surgery for any reason, migraine sufferers should be cautioned that the mandatory fasting required for surgery coupled with the anaesthetic may cause migraine pain in addition to the post-operative pain caused by the surgical procedure. It is important to inform the surgeon and anesthetist of any past history of migraine.

When no triggers can be found

Despite their best efforts, some migraine sufferers will be unable to identify their triggers. Some find that they enter periods when their migraine seems to 'flare up'. Many try to no avail to find something to attribute it to (weather, deadlines at work, etc.). If this is your experience, take heart. Some researchers believe that migraine can worsen or lessen over time as part of its natural pattern. Termed 'neuronal periodicity', this phenomenon is not completely understood, but knowing about it can bring peace of mind to those who seem to enter bad bouts for no apparent reason.

The effect of aerobic exercise on migraine

An important part of becoming healthy involves improving one's overall fitness level. A 1992 study published in the journal *Headache* showed that regular attendance at aerobics classes significantly decreased the pain of migraine attacks. There was also a trend towards reduction in the frequency and duration of the attacks experienced by the people in the study.

Regular aerobic exercise raises the body's level of endorphins, natural painkilling substances that will be on hand to battle the next attack. As well, exercise tones up the blood vessels involved with the migraine attack. And, finally, improving physical health leads to a longer, healthier, happier life and to the reduction of stress, the alleviation of depression and an improved overall sense of well-being.

Aerobic exercise does not necessarily have to mean an intense aerobics class or mountain climbing. Always start your regime slowly, and under a doctor's supervision, especially if you've spent a little too much time on the couch in recent years. An excellent aerobic schedule for migraine sufferers may involve *brisk* walking for 20 to 30 minutes, 3 or 4 times per week. Allow sufficient time for a proper warm-up and cool-down period – going at it too hard too quickly may bring on an exertional headache.

Stretching exercises are very helpful, especially if you sit at a desk or are confined to one position most of the day. Change your position and take a stretch every 20 minutes.

At the first signs of an attack, some people find that gentle aerobic exercise will actually help stop an attack from progressing. Researchers theorize that the beneficial effects come from a positive boost to blood flow. Others report that sexual activity resulting in orgasm during the early stages of a migraine can help curtail an attack. However, sex is not a universal prescription for migraine relief. Although some sufferers will experience an increase in sexual desire as a premonitory symptom before their attack, others can't even bear to be touched.

Some types of exercise may spell trouble for migraineurs. Activities that involve prolonged head-down bending or stooping may have to be avoided. Whatever exercise is chosen should be enjoyable and fit in well with the sufferer's schedule (such as riding a bicycle to work). The important thing is to stick to it. Exercise should become part of your way of life. It should also be affordable, and it is usually more fun if the activities are shared by family members and friends.

Coupled with exercise, relaxation is important, and a healthy balance between exercise and rest. Relaxation techniques should be studied by migraine sufferers to help them achieve this balance and deal with the pain when it occurs. Many techniques can be explored. See Chapter 12, 'Complementary Therapies', for more information.

Migraine in the workplace

An estimated 18 million workdays are lost in the UK each year as a result of migraine. Many other migraine sufferers may be at their desks but functioning at less than optimum levels.

Migraine is often misunderstood, and most misunderstandings seem to occur in the workplace. People frequently report a lack of sympathy from colleagues and bosses alike when migraine strikes. Many are afraid to admit the nature of their illness for fear of being disbelieved. Those in positions of authority or higher responsibility may not admit to suffering from migraine as they imagine they will appear weak, unable to 'handle stress', or, at worst, neurotic. Migraine is rarely something one would feel comfortable discussing in a job interview. Joan Didion writes in her landmark book, *The White Album*: '"Do you have headaches sometimes? frequently? never?" the application forms would demand. "Check one". Wary of the trap, wanting whatever it was that the successful circumnavigation of that particular form could bring (a job, a scholarship, the respect of mankind and the grace of God), I would check one. "Sometimes", I would lie.' Nevertheless, shoving migraine into the closet or pretending to have a more acceptable illness will not make the difficulties migraine sufferers encounter in the workplace go away.

The treatment of migraine in the workplace may be thought of as a two-step process. The goals are:

1. to raise the understanding of the serious nature of migraine among co-workers and bosses
2. to create a workplace environment that allows the sufferer to eliminate as many migraine triggers as possible (thereby reducing the number of attacks experienced, reducing absenteeism and increasing productivity).

To attain goal number one, the migraine sufferer must think of him- or herself as a spokesperson for migraine. Start by educating co-workers gradually through informal discussions (which may begin something like: 'Did you hear about the recent developments in migraine ... ?'). Sharing books or literature with others in the workplace will go a long way toward raising the understanding of migraine as the biological disorder that it is. For those who doubt, simply seeing the cover of a migraine information book or pamphlet may leave them thinking, 'Hmm, it seems there is something to this migraine thing.' In some companies, occupational health departments may be able to help organize information-sharing sessions on migraine. These may be as simple as a fifteen-minute coffee or tea break with a small group during which literature about migraine is passed around and people are asked to think for a moment about how their lives would be affected by recurring attacks of migraine. In any case, the goal is not to set the migraine sufferer up as an invalid, but to surround him or her with understanding and support. You wouldn't expect a flower to bloom in the cold of winter, so how can you expect a migraine sufferer to flourish in an unfriendly workplace?

The second goal is one that migraine sufferers reach largely under their own steam. It involves taking action to create as trigger-free an environment as possible. Here are some tips sufferers have shared over the years on reducing triggers associated with desk work at the office:

1. *Minimize eyestrain* by ensuring that surroundings are well lit. Many sufferers report fluorescent lighting to be harsh and irritating. Unfortunately, fluorescent bulbs light most workplaces and schools and usually can't be replaced by other lighting. Although manufacturers of fluorescent tubes designed to emulate natural sunlight say that full-spectrum tubes will reduce headaches, this has never been conclusively proven in all cases. Owing to the expense of this replacement and the lack of a guarantee, this is not usually a practical option. Some people report receiving relief by 'overriding' the fluorescent lighting by placing a standard desk lamp with an incandescent (non-fluorescent) bulb on their desk, even if the fluorescent tubes above must be left on.

   A study in Britain involved having 20 schoolchildren with migraine wear tinted glasses for four months whenever they were under fluorescent lighting. Children fitted with blue-tinted glasses initially responded with as great an improvement as the children who were fitted with rose-tinted glasses. After a period of four months, however, the children fitted with rose-tinted glasses were the only ones who exhibited sustained improvement. The average number of attacks experienced by the children wearing rose-tinted glasses dropped substantially, and three of the 20 children studied stopped having migraine attacks altogether. The results were scientifically validated by the fact that the rose-tinted glasses were capable of reducing visually provoked electrical activity on electroencepahalograph (EEG) testing. The researchers feared that the children would be teased for wearing the glasses, but the fashion statement caught on, and the glasses were a hit. Optical departments of many stores carry such glasses, and the least expensive pairs probably work as well as the designer ones.

Flashing or flickering lights can be quite bothersome to migraine sufferers; prolonged exposure should be avoided when possible. Migraine sufferers who spend time at a computer screen may wish to minimize eyestrain by adjusting the contrast and brightness dials on their monitor screen to the most comfortable levels. If the option is open to try other types of monitors, colour screens with green type are preferred by most. Antiglare screens are commercially available and are a matter of personal preference, but worth exploring. They can usually be tried out at computer outlets.

2. *Keep the blood flowing* throughout the body and help improve the tone of migraine-sensitive blood vessels by changing your physical position every twenty minutes or so. Although a formal break is not necessary, it's a good idea to get up out of the chair. It may be enough simply to make the next phone call while standing at the desk. Stretching out the neck and shoulders every couple of

hours will prevent tension from building up and acting as a trigger. Consider keeping a mirror in your desk so that you can monitor your facial expression every so often. What you should see is a relaxed, friendly face. If that's not what's shining back in the mirror, smiling and relaxing the jaw will stop the muscles of the face from triggering a headache.

3. *Avoid the food triggers* of migraine in the workplace; it is usually easily accomplished by bringing lunch from home. Fast food and cafeteria fare often contain migraine-triggering food additives, and the selection is often limited. Taking the extra few minutes to pack lunch and snack foods can reduce migraine attacks (and increase pocket money).

4. *Optimize physical fitness*. This is a key element to anyone's plan to reduce migraine and is especially important to people who work outside the home. Occupations that involve a minimal amount of physical exertion can leave workers unfit and lead to higher levels of stress, anxiety and depression as the body's level of endorphins drops during non-activity. This is especially true in the cold, dark winter months when many office employees find their activity reduced to rushing from warm home to office and back, with evenings spent on the living-room sofa. The end result may be an increase in migraine attacks. Making use of any company fitness facilities is a good start. Join a gym or sign up for swimming or aerobics classes. Taking a brisk walk at lunch (yes, even in the cold) is an excellent habit and is best enjoyed in the company of others from the office (a good time to bring a little migraine education into the conversation, too).

Being an advocate for fitness is contagious and may lead to increased productivity in the workplace for all.

5. *Stop the overuse of pain relievers* and seek out all available migraine-specific treatment options and non-drug treatment strategies. This technique is of utmost importance for all migraine sufferers. Migraine can be managed in and out of the workplace only when sufferers take action for themselves.

Migraine at home

Since migraine affects sufferers at work and at home, it creates certain challenges around the home. Women and men who are at home raising a family don't have the option to call in sick. They also frequently do not have the support of workplace programmes, colleagues, sickness benefits, or other employee support programmes. Women and men who balance full- or part-time employment outside of the home with the full-time job of raising a family have the challenge of managing migraine in two workplaces – the office and the home – while arranging for and monitoring care-givers at the same time. But the time and effort spent maintaining migraine-prevention strategies will lead to better health and control of migraine than simply reaching for a bottle of pain relievers when the first twinges of an attack occur.

In addition to the other 'getting healthy' strategies mentioned in this chapter so far, here are some tips for migraine sufferers at home:

1. *Develop household routines* for housework, shopping and cooking. Getting into a pattern will help everyone in the

home to stay organized. Partners and children will get used to putting out the dustbins on a certain night, or hoovering every other Saturday, for example. Getting a jump start on the next morning before going to bed will help to reduce commotion in the morning (try making lunches and laying out clothes before going to bed). Making an effort to stay reasonably on top of things will pay off if migraine strikes and renders you unavailable for a time. If there is at least *something* for the family to throw together for supper and something clean to wear, it will give you relative peace of mind when you get a migraine.

2. *Consider purchasing non-harsh cleaning products.* The 'environmentally friendly' cleaners that are emerging are usually free of ammonia and other strong-smelling chemicals. The strong odours of some of these products really get some heads pounding. Migraine sufferers do well to invest, when possible, in self-cleaning ovens, and to buy long-handled mops and other cleaning tools to avoid prolonged bending or stooping, which can send blood rushing to the pain-sensitive blood vessels in the head.

A light-blocking blind on the bedroom window and a 'Quiet – Headache in Progress' sign for the bedroom door should be standard equipment. Partners can help during severe attacks by taking charge of the phone, reducing noise around the house (headphones for stereos are a good investment), preparing meals and lending support in general. Many sufferers report wanting their own space to a certain extent, but at the same time wanting to know that loved ones are close by and checking in frequently. Dropping by the bedroom with a fresh icepack and a damp towel for the forehead brings relief to someone in the throes of an attack. Check Chapter 11's suggestions for comfort measures to see what else can be offered to ease the discomfort of an attack in progress. However, *just being there* is heaven-sent help to a migraine sufferer.

8
Medical Treatment of Migraine Attacks

Contrary to popular belief and common practice, the proper first step in the treatment of migraine does *not* involve reaching for a pill. Our society expects there to be a pill for every illness and great lengths are taken by some to find the 'magic cure' – the silver bullet that will take away all the pain. We can put a man on the moon, but there are only slightly more than a couple of dozen illnesses that are curable through the use of pharmaceutical preparations. Headache is not one of them.

Realistically speaking, the goal of migraine therapy is to achieve maximum control over the number of attacks experienced and to relieve as much as possible the symptoms of the attacks that do occur. Most often the best relief is found by preventing the start of attacks through the identification and elimination (where possible) of trigger factors and by optimizing personal levels of physical and mental health. For many, these first two measures will go a long way in reducing (or even eliminating, for a lucky few) the number of attacks.

However, for most migraine sufferers, recurring migraine requires taking treatment action. Although the ultimate goal may be to control migraine without the use of medication, the treatment of migraine often involves the safe and sensible use of prescription or non-prescription drugs (sometimes both) at one time or another.

The following discussion of particular medications does not include a complete description of the action, side effects or contraindications of any of the drugs, nor does it say which (if any) are best for any one person. Anyone seeking pharmaceutical relief from migraine must consult a physician about suitable medications and should report back to the doctor so that responses and any side effects can be properly monitored and managed. It is the patient's responsibility to report any side effects (whether expected or not) to a physician without delay. Fortunately, most people experience few or no side effects from their medications. There is no one medication that will work or is suitable for everyone. Responses to medication will also vary.

Medications are in most cases referred to by their generic (chemical) names. For examples of some available brands, see the Table of Drug Names at the end of the book.

Researchers and patients generally agree that the following properties (in no particular order) would make for a perfect migraine drug:

- completely effective at relieving pain and other symptoms for all who take it
- quick acting
- easy to administer
- free from side effects
- non-sedating
- non-addictive

- unlikely to cause medication-induced headache
- unlikely to cause headache recurrence after successful treatment
- inexpensive.

No drug yet exists that meets all these criteria. But it is worth the effort to be diligent in finding medication with the *best* qualities and effects for you. Most migraine sufferers will try many different medications throughout their lifetime, and some say they feel as if they are being treated like a guinea pig. Nevertheless, physicians who are willing to try different medications and work in partnership with their patients in monitoring responses have the patients' best interests in mind. If both doctor and patient persist, sooner or later the best treatment, or combination of treatments, will be found.

Migraine sufferers live in anticipation of the next new migraine medication or other treatment. Whether they are trying a medication that is new to them or a medication that is new on the market, some have become afraid to be overly optimistic. Some medications will help; others won't. Some medications will work fabulously at the beginning but somehow lose their effectiveness over time. The drug that helps one attack may not help all attacks as effectively; still other medications will cause unacceptable side effects. Some sufferers will flatly refuse to even try a medication because of the effect or lack of effect it had on a friend or family member. But it is important to retain a degree of optimism when considering new therapies. Individual response is the biggest factor in drug therapy. Promising results from scientific research indicate what most will experience, but nobody knows whether he or she will be part of the majority until the treatment is tried personally.

A universally safe and effective therapy is not yet available, and there is no cure for migraine. Therefore, the goal of therapy may be to prevent attacks from ever starting. Medication may be used to prevent particularly severe or disabling attacks. The use of preventive techniques or therapies is sometimes referred to as 'prophylactic' therapy. For attacks that break through despite your best efforts at prevention, the goal of therapy may be adequate symptom relief, often using medication, once the attack is in progress. In any case, it is important for those prone to migraine to adopt realistic expectations of their medicines and the doctors who prescribe them. If migraine sufferers walk into a doctor's office and expect the doctor to scribble a prescription for a cure-all, they are unlikely to find relief. Patients who take responsibility for being the managers of their own migraine have a much better chance of finding real relief. This involves recognizing that their migraines are theirs to keep (at least for now) and theirs to control, and it involves consulting a doctor for help on what they can do in partnership to bring their migraine under control. This is the cornerstone for the effective treatment of migraine.

The study and practice of complementary therapies may eventually reduce or eliminate the need for medications for some. Subsequent chapters will examine complementary or 'alternative' options that may be initiated before the use of medication, in combination with any medications tried, or when medications fail to provide adequate relief.

Medication for symptomatic relief

Two main types of medications are used for the treatment of migraines. The first is medication to combat the symptoms of a migraine once it is in progress. This is known as 'medication for symptomatic relief'. The second is specialized medication given daily to help prevent migraine attacks from ever starting. This is known as 'preventive (prophylactic) medication'. We will now look at the first type of medication – medication for symptomatic relief.

To give medications their best chance to work, migraine sufferers should take time out to rest immediately after taking their medicine, if possible. This rest period will give the medicine time to start working and will help the sufferer to regroup. An hour is the preferred length of time, but a rest period of even 15 minutes may prove helpful. As well, symptomatic medication should be taken as early on in an attack as possible.

Non-prescription pain relievers

On the shelves of every chemist's there is a section reserved for products for the relief of pain and headache. You can also find an assortment of pain relievers on the shelf at the grocery shop. Television advertisements tell us of the benefits of readily available pain-relieving preparations. It is no wonder, then, that many migraine sufferers treat their pain with these preparations before ever consulting a doctor. Most do it believing they have a so-called tension headache. Indeed, these preparations may be all that sufferers of occasional tension-type headache will ever need and they may offer good relief to those with minor discomfort. But, in the case of migraine, these medications are frequently ineffective. And overuse of them can make the symptoms of migraine worse through medication-induced headache or analgesic-withdrawal headache. Nevertheless, the frequent use of non-prescription preparations (by 91 per cent of migraine sufferers) merits mention of the most popular types used.

Of the non-prescription pain relievers available, aspirin is the oldest. Aspirin's pain-relieving properties are believed to result from its ability to inactivate an enzyme necessary for the production of prostaglandins. Prostaglandins are pain-producing substances found in the body. Aspirin is also a useful anti-inflammatory in higher doses (the anti-inflammatory effect is due to inhibition of prostaglandins) and it can act to bring down a fever. Taken early in a migraine attack, at adequate dose levels, aspirin can be helpful for some in reducing the pain. It should not be taken by people with certain health problems such as aspirin-sensitive asthma, peptic ulcers or bleeding disorders. In recent years, the use of aspirin in children with certain illnesses (notably chicken pox and influenza) has been linked to the often fatal Reye's syndrome. Aspirin has the potential to cause side effects in some, most commonly irritation of the lining of the stomach. Recent studies hail aspirin as a wonder drug. Its anti-platelet activities make it a suitable treatment for reducing the risk of heart attack in some people. Some doctors recommend that some patients use small amounts of aspirin for the prevention of migraine attacks, but this program should be tried only on the advice of a physician.

Paracetamol is a very popular pain reliever. Many products contain paracetamol. Studies show it has pain-relieving and anti-fever capabilities equal to those of aspirin, although it is considered less effective for migraine than aspirin or ibuprofen. Unlike aspirin, however, it is not an anti-inflammatory or anti-platelet agent. Paracetamol has an advantage for some over aspirin in that it is less likely to cause stomach upset. Both paracetamol and aspirin are available in 'extra strength' formulations, which are simply a higher dose of medication (usually 500 milligrams or more, versus the regular-strength dose of 325 milligrams). Used as directed, paracetamol will be unlikely to cause adverse effects. Paracetamol may be used during pregnancy under the direct supervision and advice of a doctor.

More recently, ibuprofen has been added to the list of readily available pain relievers. Ibuprofen is a non-steroidal anti-inflammatory agent. Its ability to reduce pain is believed to stem from its ability to block the production of pain-producing prostaglandins. It can also bring down fever. Although not suitable for people with a history of inflammatory stomach problems or ulcers, ibuprofen has been found to be less likely to cause gastrointestinal bleeding at normal doses than is aspirin. Ibuprofen should not be used by people with aspirin-sensitive asthma.

To avoid medication-induced headache, do not take any pain reliever more often than directed, or on more than three days per week. It is probably a good idea to have the approval of a doctor before taking any over-the-counter preparations regularly. If pain relievers are required as often as two or three times per week, migraine-specific treatments should be considered. It is easy for the use of pain relievers to move rapidly from this level to a higher, unacceptable level.

Of relevance to migraine sufferers are the preparations containing small amounts of codeine. Used judiciously, these preparations can provide relief from mild to moderate migraine pain. But overuse of codeine-containing preparations can result in stubborn medication-induced headaches.

Non-prescription anti-nausea preparations

The anti-nausea and anti-vomiting medication domperidone is found in non-prescription preparations. Since migraine is

Caffeine

Although not thought of by most people as a drug, caffeine may act as an analgesic in headache. Many swear by a cup of espresso or strong coffee (with or without their symptomatic medications) at the onset of a migraine to stave off a full-blown attack. Some argue that this boost of caffeine corrects a caffeine-withdrawal headache, while others say caffeine can act as a vasoconstrictor and ward off a migraine. Caffeine is added to many off-the-shelf, over-the-counter and prescription pain relievers for these reasons: it increases gastric secretions and helps the stomach to empty and it is a stimulant that may help to counteract some of the drowsiness caused by certain pain relievers.

often associated with nausea, vomiting or both, domperidone is a useful preparation for some. It cannot be used by men with an enlarged prostate gland. It is available as a pill, liquid or suppository, in adult and paediatric doses.

Non-prescription sinus and cold remedies

The symptoms of migraine are frequently confused with the symptoms of sinus headache. True sinus headache is usually accompanied by fever, nasal discharge and other such evidence of infection. Many people who believe they are suffering from sinus headache are actually suffering from migraine pain in the face or sinus area. The relief obtained from 'sinus medication' may result largely from the aspirin or paracetamol that is often added to the sinus remedy. It is important to check with a doctor for diagnosis and proper treatment of any recurring head or face pain.

Cough and cold products containing phenylpropanolamine (ppa) must be avoided, as this agent is an independent risk factor for haemorrhagic stroke.

Prescription pain relievers

A 1990 survey showed that 44 per cent of migraine sufferers who saw a physician received prescription medication for their attacks. The most common type of prescription was for a pain reliever.

Prescription pain-relieving medications formed the mainstay of migraine treatment for a long time. They act by blanketing the painful impulses of migraine. Most people find it takes a prescription-strength pain reliever to 'break' a migraine attack. There is nothing fancy or migraine-specific about these medications, which are also used for pain from other sources.

Many have found relief through occasional use of combination analgesic preparations. However, recent knowledge of the role that frequent use of analgesics can play in the generation of medication-induced headache leading to chronic daily headache has left many physicians hesitant to prescribe pain relievers. Many prefer to recommend trying migraine-specific treatments, especially if there is a need for more than occasional use of medication.

Every day patients are being told that they will no longer be receiving the usual painkillers for migraine. Many are led to believe that the doctor's unwillingness to prescribe the painkiller stems from the belief that the patient has become or is likely to become 'addicted' to the drug. In fact, addiction to pain relievers is rare among headache patients. The real reason for discouraging the use of pain relievers on more than an occasional basis is rebound or medication-induced headache. (See Chapter 3 for a detailed discussion of this type of headache, which is actually caused by the overuse of pain relievers.) Another factor in the new line of thinking among doctors is the availability of migraine-specific treatments that may be more suitable to the disorder. Because there are other options than simply blanketing the pain of migraine, doctors are able to offer their patients non-narcotic solutions. If, however, your doctor simply stops prescribing the pain reliever and tells you to go home and live with the pain, look for another doctor who will work with you to explore migraine medications that can help you control your migraine while avoiding the overuse of pain relievers. Don't turn from your prescription pain relievers to large quantities of over-the-counter ones. You'll only feel worse in the end.

Prescription tranquillizers, sedatives, anti-anxiety agents and sleeping pills

In days of old, many migraine sufferers were prescribed 'nerve pills' in the belief that their headaches were caused by stress. Stress is not the *cause* of migraine; however, the biochemical processes behind the physical disorder of migraine can be kicked off by the *trigger* of stress. Also, the pain associated with migraine attacks can evoke a level of anxiety; hence, the addition of small amounts of sedatives to some prescription-only combination pain relievers used in migraine. But taking medication prescribed for anxiety as part of the treatment of migraine is apt to do more harm than good. These compounds (which also include sleeping pills and non-prescription sleep aids) may cause an increase in any depression present, and are likely to interfere with normal sleep patterns. The use of these medications for the treatment of migraine is not recommended.

Prescription anti-inflammatories

Non-steroidal anti-inflammatory drugs (NSAIDs) may be used to treat an attack in progress or as a preventive agent to help reduce the number of attacks. The side effects they can cause are similar to those caused by aspirin. It is best to take these medications with food to lessen the possibility of stomach irritation. NSAIDs such as naproxen or naproxen sodium are sometimes given around the time of the menstrual period to reduce the occurrence of menstrual migraine in susceptible women. Other non-steroidal anti-inflammatory drugs include flurbiprofen, diclofenac sodium, and keto-profen.

Indomethacin is a type of non-steroidal anti-inflammatory that is almost universally effective for certain specific headache syndromes. The diagnosis of paroxysmal hemi-crania and hemicrania continua is confirmed if the symp-toms of these syndromes respond to treatment with indomethacin. This medication is often also used to treat benign exertional and cough headaches, sex headaches and idiopathic stabbing headache (see Chapter 3 for descriptions of these headache syndromes), but its effectiveness is not diagnostic of these problems.

Ketorolac tromethamine is a non-steroidal anti-inflam-matory drug. It can be given in pill form for mild to moderate pain or by injection for moderate to severe pain or when nausea or vomiting is present.

Prescription anti-nausea preparations

During a migraine, the stomach does not empty properly, and medication taken once an attack is in progress is not absorbed well. For this reason, medications that enhance gastric emptying such as metoclopramide hydrochloride or domperidone maleate may be prescribed to be taken before pain relievers to facilitate in the absorption of the pain reliever. The nausea believed to be a result of the stomach's inability to empty may be relieved through the use of gastric-motility enhancers. In addition, although further evidence is needed, some believe that domperidone (given on its own in the early stages of an attack) may stop a migraine from progressing because of certain chemical properties of the drug.

Prescription migraine-specific symptomatic medications

The notion that it is better to address the symptoms of migraine at the root cause rather than simply numbing the pain with a pain reliever has led to the treatment of migraine with migraine-specific medication.

Ergotamine tartrate has been used since the 1920s to shrink blood vessels around the brain that become swollen during a migraine. Ergotamine also has an effect on the

Bread and the Devil

Ergotamine is derived from a fungus called *Claviceps purpurea* that grows naturally on rye. If large amounts of rye fungus are eaten (or if too much ergotamine is taken), psychiatric hallucinations and gangrene can result. There have been reports of outbreaks of mental illness, and gangrene in the hands and feet, among people who ate bread made from rotting rye. In the past, the mental illness was known as St Anthony's fire, which people believed was caused by a visit from the devil to their village. Those afflicted were cured of their hallucinations and burning hands and feet by visiting St Anthony's shrine, which was located in another village. The rye crops surrounding the village of St Anthony's shrine were not infected by fungal growth, so their symptoms dissipated.

serotonin pathway that is now believed to have a role in the generation of migraine pain.

Ergotamine-containing preparations must be taken at the first sign of an attack. The most common side effects experienced by some include nausea. For this reason, some ergotamine compounds also contain domperidone to combat the nausea. Quite often, however, the nausea will still occur. Other compounds combine ergotamine with caffeine, some have belladonna added to help with any excessive nausea and vomiting, and pentobarbital is added to some although no effective role for this addition has been shown. Ergotamine preparations and their derivatives should not be taken by pregnant or breastfeeding women or by people who have other health conditions that would make constriction of the blood vessels or a reduction in blood flow a problem (such as heart disease, history of heart attack, high blood pressure, vascular disease, angina, or kidney problems).

Ergotamine preparations are available as tablets, as tiny pills that are dissolved under the tongue (sublingual pills) and as suppositories. An ergot derivative known as dihydro-ergotamine mesylate, or DHE, is available as an injection and as a nasal spray. DHE can be effective in stopping prolonged or exceptionally severe attacks, particularly when there is an element of rebound involved. For this reason, many emergency departments are now using DHE to break long attacks instead of using traditional narcotics that may add to the rebound effect. DHE injections (in particular) may cause nausea and vomiting. Many doctors will give an anti-nausea drug such as metoclopramide hydrochloride before administering the DHE by injection. (Since metoclopramide may relieve the attack on its own, often the doctor will proceed with the DHE administration only if it is still necessary.)

Users of ergotamine must be careful to monitor themselves

to avoid overuse of the drug. Ergotamines must be used only as directed by the physician. Generally speaking, the doctor will likely recommend that, to avoid toxic effects, no more than 6 milligrams of ergotamine be taken on any particular day. Furthermore, no more than 10 milligrams of ergotamine should be taken in any particular week and no more than 20 milligrams should ever be taken in any particular month. Perhaps as important, since ergotamine can perpetuate the cycle of rebound headache in the same way that pain relievers can, ergotamine should never be taken on more than two days in any particular week. With the advent of newer medications, ergotamine's role in migraine today is limited.

At toxic levels, ergotamines can cause gangrene in the fingers and toes. 'Ergotism' is the medical term used to describe the collection of symptoms that can result from the overuse of ergot. Symptoms of ergotism include:

- nausea and vomiting
- swollen fingers
- leg or heel cramps, especially when walking
- blue colour to lower limbs on both sides
- cold fingers or toes
- abdominal pain.

Anyone experiencing any of these symptoms while taking ergotamine compounds should report to the doctor at once. The overuse of ergot tends to cause nausea, vomiting and rebound headache more commonly than circulatory problems in the fingers and toes.

Ergotamine is chemically related to the hallucinogen lysergic acid diethylamide (LSD), which explains its ability to cause hallucinations at toxic levels. Dr Albert Hofmann first synthesized LSD in his laboratory in 1943 when working with ergot fungus in a search for more effective migraine preparations. When some of the chemical was absorbed through the skin of his fingers, he began to suffer what he describes as a 'horrible terrible, terrible experience'. Hofmann calls LSD his 'problem child'. (LSD was never used for the treatment of migraine.)

For most people, the triptan group of medicines (see Chapter 9) will be preferred over ergotamines as there are fewer side effects and the triptans are associated with greater effectiveness in general. However, ergotamines are less expensive.

A medication called isometheptene mucate is often used in combination with the pain reliever paracetamol to treat a migraine attack. Isometheptene mucate is a blood-vessel constrictor and products containing it are sometimes selected for use in children (although studies have been done only in adult patients) and in people who don't tolerate ergotamine well.

9
The Triptans

In the last ten years there has been a revolution in our understanding of acute migraine attacks and our ability to treat them. Imaging has shown that there is an area at the back of the brain, in the brain stem, that becomes active at the beginning of an attack. The trigeminal nucleus, the part of the main nerve that deals with sensation in the head, becomes activated and impulses are sent backwards along nerve fibres that usually conduct impulses to the nucleus from the structures that generate sensation. These impulses cause the release of substances around the blood vessels, which make them inflamed and dilated. What is exciting is that it is now known that, when activated, certain receptors around these blood vessels and in the nerves around the blood vessels *block this action altogether*. The dilation of the blood vessels is blocked, and so is the release of inflammation-causing substances around the blood vessels. At the same time, the impulses that arise in the trigeminal nerve nucleus can also be blocked by activating the same receptor on the nerve endings around the blood vessels. (A receptor can be thought of as a lock, which is unlocked by certain compounds.)

Sumatriptan

Sumatriptan was the first of the class of compounds known as the 'triptans' to be released. It had been the subject of a huge number of studies – indeed, more studies than had ever been done on any compound in migraine prior to this. It became apparent that sumatriptan stimulated the receptors known as 5-HT_{1B} receptors, which are on the blood vessels and cause constriction of the blood vessels, and 5-HT_{1D} receptors, which are on the nerve and cause the release of inflammatory substances. Since 5-HT (5-hydroxytryptamine) is also known as serotonin, many people erroneously think that these drugs have an effect on serotonin levels. The serotonin levels may or may not change, but what is actually happening is that a receptor which is usually 'unlocked' by serotonin is being 'unlocked' by this compound.

With the introduction of sumatriptan, many patients found relief from their headaches for the first time. The drug dihydroergotamine had been available since 1945 and was also extremely effective in treating headaches, but it had a number of troublesome side effects, although fewer than an earlier, related drug, ergotamine (for more on ergotamine see Chapter 8). For some reason dihydroergotamine had been forgotten for the next 40 years, only to be resurrected in the 1980s for use in emergency, for severe migraines and in the treatment of patients with chronic headaches that were difficult to control. It then turned out that dihydroergotamine had exactly the same activity and potency at these receptors as sumatriptan. The problem was that dihydroergotamine was active at other receptors not related to the serotonin system, which was sometimes advantageous but sometimes led to unwanted side effects.

The first trials of sumatriptan were started in the 1980s.

These were of the subcutaneous compound, which is delivered by means of an auto injector (a device that makes it easy for people to administer their own injections) and is still available. The trials showed that subcutaneous sumatriptan was an extremely effective, fast-acting drug, and it became available as a prescription in the 1990s.

Just after the start of trials for subcutaneous sumatriptan, trials began with oral sumatriptan. The drug quickly found a place in the treatment of migraine and is still the best-selling medication for migraine in the world. So far over 300 million attacks have been treated with little in the way of adverse events.

In the beginning sumatriptan was associated with a number of significant side effects – some patients developed chest pains and in a few cases heart attacks following its use – but there does not seem to have been much problem in this regard recently, possibly due to a better understanding of which patients should not use this drug. Triptans and dihydroergotamine do both have some effect on the blood vessels in the head and in the heart. Chest tightness and tightness or heaviness in the throat, neck or jaw are common side effects of most of the triptan group. As well, triptans may cause tiredness, sleepiness, nausea, tingling in the extremities and a variety of other problems such as dizziness. But these side effects do not occur in most people, and when they do occur they are often not severe and are very transitory.

Following the introduction of oral sumatriptan, it became evident that a 50-milligram dose was as effective as 100 milligrams, and was better tolerated. Intranasal sumatriptan, at 5 and 20 milligrams, has since been introduced (20 milligrams is the optimal dose). The intranasal formulation is quite effective but unfortunately some people do not like substances in their nose, and some develop a bad taste in the mouth as the preparation goes over the inside of the nose and down into the mouth. Ideally, nasal preparations are absorbed through the mucous membranes inside the nose, at the top of the nose, where the membranes are particularly thin. In practice this is difficult to achieve, and the acceptability of nasal preparations has been variable, but they may be useful for people who cannot take medications by mouth because of nausea and vomiting.

Dihydroergotamine is also available as a nasal preparation, and for some people it's a very effective drug, but others find that it causes unacceptable nasal stuffiness. In some countries sumatriptan suppositories have been available.

Naratriptan

Naratriptan has slightly different properties from the other triptans in that it has a somewhat slower time to onset and it seems to last longer – i.e., there is less chance of the headache coming back quickly. On the other hand, its overall efficacy is not as good as that of other triptans. Many patients prefer it, however, and it is especially useful if the headaches start slowly and last a long time. At present the 1-milligram dose is being studied as a preventive for menstrual migraine; it is too early to say whether this will be effective, but early studies have been encouraging. Naratriptan is available in 2.5-milligram doses. The latter is more effective and in studies it has had no more side effects than those in patients on a placebo.

Zolmitriptan

Zolmitriptan is available in the 2.5-milligram strength, and this strength appears to offer optimum efficacy with a minimum of side effects. However, some people need a slightly higher dosage, and for this reason a 5-milligram version is sometimes recommended. The onset of action is quite rapid. Side effects are very similar to those with sumatriptan. Studies have been done of zolmitriptan nasal spray, and zolmitriptan 'melt', which is a rapidly dispersible tablet with an orange taste, is just being released. Their efficacy appears to be encouraging and they are well tolerated.

Rizatriptan

Rizatriptan is available in 5- and 10-milligram doses, and in 5- and 10-milligram dispersible tablets which have a mint taste. The dissolving tablets have been shown to be very well tolerated and indeed many people prefer them to the plain tablets. They can be taken without water, so they are convenient to take anywhere, and they can be useful for someone with nausea. Rizatriptan has a similar range of side effects to both sumatriptan and zolmitriptan. It has a rapid time to onset – some studies have suggested that it is more rapid than sumatriptan or zolmitriptan – and it appears to have more effect on nausea than the other medications available.

Almotriptan

The most recently released triptan is almotriptan. A recent analysis of all the triptans confirmed that almotriptan is effective and well tolerated when compared to the other drugs in this category. It is available in 6.25- and 12.5-milligram oral tablets. Using almotriptan with medications that are metabolized via a body system called CYP450 results in increased levels of almotriptan. These include drugs such as ketoconazole (Nizoral) and quite possibly other medicines in this category such as erythromycin. Always notify your doctor and pharmacist of all medications you are taking.

Taking triptans

Thus four new medications for migraine have appeared in a relatively short time. Sumatriptan is by far the best established, and has been shown to be effective and safe over large numbers of patients in the last nine years. However, all the triptans seem to be similar in efficacy, with naratriptan being less effective but having other potentially useful properties. The decision as to which triptan to take is based on considerations such as individual response and tolerance, the characteristics of the attacks, how well symptoms other than pain are relieved, the tendency for attacks to recur, how consistently the drug works and which drug and delivery system the individual prefers.

It is fair to say, however, that overuse of medications such as triptans can lead to problems. The most common is the rebound or medication-induced headache: headaches may start coming back as soon as the medication wears off. It is unwise to use more than about 18 tablets of these medications in a month. If the headaches are more frequent than that, another approach needs to be taken, such as using preventive medications.

It may be worth discussing the way medications are assessed and used in clinical trials. For the sake of simplicity, headaches have been subdivided into four categories: 'severe', 'moderate', 'mild' or 'none'. To determine whether a patient has responded to a medication, one looks to see whether he or she has moved from the 'severe' or 'moderate' category to the 'mild' or 'none' category. The usual timeframe is two hours, although in more recent trials an effort has been made to look at responses earlier than this.

Of course, people would rather not have a headache at all, and would prefer that 'pain-free' be the final measure. In practice, however, it is useful to look at reduction of the headache to 'mild', since this allows the person to continue day-to-day activities without too much hindrance. If we fix our hopes on a magically pain-free result, the success rate may be low and the drug may seem disappointing.

People who do not respond particularly well to one of the triptans, or do not tolerate one, should certainly try another, and if necessary a third one. Studies have shown that if the response to the first medication is poor there is a 75 per cent chance of a good response to the second one and a 15 per cent chance of a good response to the third one. Overall, the triptans benefit at least 70–80 per cent of patients, and they have had a dramatic impact on quality of life in numerous people who had previously been disabled by their migraines.

Nevertheless, there are people for whom this class of medication does not work, or in whom it should not be used. You should not use triptans if you have a history of heart disease, angina, high blood pressure or other circulatory problems.

Some people choose not to use triptans because of adverse events such as chest tightness, throat tightness and feelings of tiredness, and have to use more traditional forms of treatment. Triptans are not the last word in migraine medication. Other areas are being actively explored by the pharmaceutical industry. No doubt, by the time this book reaches another edition, there will be many more medications available to treat migraine.

10
Preventive and Emergency Treatment

Many people are able to treat their migraine successfully by first eliminating the controllable triggers; improving their physical, mental and emotional health; and treating the symptoms of any remaining attacks with non-drug strategies. Many rely on the occasional use of pain relievers or migraine-specific medications for attacks in progress. For others, migraine is more of a challenge to control.

Those who experience three or more migraines per month, or who experience varieties of migraine with dramatic symptoms, such as basilar migraine, may wish to consider preventive therapy with medications. Known medically as 'prophylactic therapy', this is a regimen where specific types of medications are taken every day (whether there is a headache present or not) to right the biochemical imbalance that underpins migraine. The intended result is to decrease the frequency, intensity or duration of migraine attacks. Preventive medications are not pain relievers. Preventive medications are often taken in small doses and their potential to cause side effects may be less troublesome than the overuse of painkilling or symptomatic medications. Preventives take time to begin working. Therapy is usually continued for four to twelve months without interruption, then is tapered down or stopped for a period of evaluation. In many cases, the benefits received while taking the medication will continue for a time after use of the drug is stopped. The migraine itself may enter a period of less activity or near-remission, or the break may be a residual effect of the medication.

Some people find that, after a time, their body gets used to the preventive medication they are on, and the drug stops working. In this case, it is best to speak to the doctor about stopping the drug for a while and perhaps switching to another. Most people then find that, after a period, they can retry the original medication and it will begin to work again.

Despite the proven effectiveness of preventive therapy for many, only about 6 per cent of migraine sufferers were found in a 1990 survey to be taking daily preventive medicine. Some experts cite as an explanation the general lack of knowledge regarding the use of these medications in migraine; others believe some people may be reluctant to take medication daily even though it can substantially reduce the total consumption of pain relievers or other symptomatic medicines. Other factors may include side effects and cost; also, with the availability of the triptans, some people may have less need for preventive drugs.

Beta-adrenergic blockers

Most prophylactic medications were originally developed to treat other disorders, and were discovered, through serendipity, also to be helpful in migraine. This is true of beta blockers. These medicines, which were developed to treat high blood pressure, were found to help reduce the number of migraines experienced by patients who also suffered from migraine. No one really knows how beta blockers work in migraine, but they have been shown to be helpful time and time again in clinical trials. They are the oldest and most widely used migraine preventive today. Common beta blockers used for the preventive treatment of migraine include propranolol; the oldest, nadolol, sometimes favoured because of the lower incidence of certain side effects; timolol maleate; atenolol; and metoprolol. A recent European study indicates that adding therapeutic riboflavin to beta-blocker therapy may increase the effectiveness of the treatment.

Beta blockers may be a good choice for migraine prevention if high blood pressure also exists, since one drug can treat both conditions. They should not be used by people who suffer from asthma, diabetes or certain heart problems. When it is time to stop taking beta blockers, use must be decreased gradually to prevent problems such as heart palpitations, high blood pressure and a worsening of headaches. Potential side effects of beta blockers include a slower heartbeat, stomach upset, sleep disturbances or a reduction or loss of libido (sex drive). They should be used only with caution in people with depression, and it should be noted that beta blockers can limit athletic performance.

Calcium-channel blockers

Like beta blockers, most calcium-channel blockers (except for flunarizine) were originally developed to treat certain heart problems. They too were coincidentally found to reduce the number of migraines experienced by some. Calcium-channel blockers are believed to work by stabilizing blood vessels through preventing them from either constricting (narrowing) or dilating (widening). The calcium-channel blocker verapamil is commonly used for the prevention of cluster headache. They do not cause a depletion of calcium in the body and will not cause osteoporosis. Migraine is not caused by an excess of calcium, and sufferers need not limit their calcium intake to avoid migraine or supplement their calcium intake while taking a calcium-channel blocker.

Calcium-channel blockers take longer to begin to work, and may take up to two months to reach their peak effect. They too carry potential side effects and contraindications. Constipation is one of the most frequently reported side effects of verapamil. They are not suitable for people with certain types of heart disease. Commonly used calcium-channel blockers include verapamil and diltiazem.

A special form of calcium-channel blocker was developed for use specifically in migraine. Flunarizine was designed to act only on the blood vessels of the head and it does not have the heart effects that the regular calcium-channel blockers do. However, it should not be used by people with a history of depression. Like its calcium-channel-blocking relatives, it can cause weight gain and drowsiness, among other side effects.

Non-steroidal anti-inflammatories (NSAIDs)

Examples of these medicines include ibuprofen, naproxen and naproxen sodium, and more information about them can be found in Chapter 8. In this chapter, however, NSAIDs need to be considered for their ability to act as preventive medications – especially when taken around the time of the menstrual period during the headache-prone days. It is *very* important to embark on this daily use of NSAIDs only under a doctor's supervision, as taking NSAIDs excessively – even over-the-counter ones such as ibuprofen – can lead to stomach irritation.

Antidepressants

Another class of prophylactic migraine medications has caused many misunderstandings between doctors and their patients. Antidepressants (used to treat depression) are often used for migraine prevention. They are often prescribed for migraine at smaller doses than would be used to treat depression. Antidepressants are helpful to some people with migraine as their chemical action helps to correct the chemical imbalances behind the migraine disorder. They also have pain-relieving properties and are used for general pain relief in a variety of painful disorders. Misunderstanding will arise, however, if the patient does not understand why an antidepressant is being used for the treatment of pain. Uninformed migraine patients often think that the doctor secretly believes them to be depressed and doesn't really understand migraine. Although depression can certainly accompany migraine and has been shown to be more prevalent in migraine sufferers (migraine is also more prevalent in people with depression), most often the antidepressant is not being used to treat depression when prescribed for migraine prevention.

Tricyclic antidepressants (sometimes referred to as tricyclic analgesics) commonly used for the treatment of migraine are amitriptyline, nortriptyline and doxepin. Tricyclic antidepressants are contraindicated for use by people with some types of glaucoma, epilepsy or heart-rhythm disturbances, or by men with enlargement of the prostate. Dryness of the mouth is a common side effect. The potential ability of tricyclic antidepressants to cause sedation is less of a problem if the medication is taken at bedtime or slightly earlier in the evening.

The newer class of antidepressants known as SSRIs (selective serotonin reuptake inhibitors) is sometimes used for migraine prevention – especially if a mood disorder exists. Examples of SSRIs include fluoxetine, fluvoxamine, citalopram, paroxetine and sertraline. They are considered to be less effective than the tricyclics. Headache can occur as a side effect to SSRIs but it often goes away over time.

Further studies of other drugs originally used for the treatment of psychiatric disorders, such as the MAO (monoamine oxidase, an enzyme) inhibitor phenelzine sulfate, are needed to tell us if they have any value in the treatment of migraine. MAOs are rarely used for migraine. (Interestingly, people who take MAO inhibitors must stick to a diet low in tyramine to avoid a serious drug reaction. Since migraine sufferers also benefit from a diet low in tyramine – a vasoactive substance believed to trigger migraine and present in foods such as mature cheese, red wine, pickled herring, etc. – many believe that the benefits of MAO-inhibitor therapy in migraine stem from the diet, not the drug.) MAO inhibitors should not be taken in combination with SSRIs, medicines for colds, some pain relievers or certain other medications used to treat migraine. Check carefully with the doctor or chemist.

Antiserotonin agents

Probably one of the most effective preventive agents for migraine is methysergide maleate. It belongs to a group of medicines called 'ergot alkaloids'. First introduced in 1959, it was shown in one study to reduce headaches by more than 50 per cent in 90 per cent of patients. However, its use today is generally reserved for severe, persistent migraine because it can produce more serious side effects if used on a prolonged basis. A condition known as 'retroperitoneal fibrosis', characterized by the formation of fibrous tissue around vital organs in the abdomen or chest, may result if methysergide is taken for longer than four to six months at a time. Patients taking methysergide are monitored with yearly radiological tests to watch for the formation of this fibrous tissue.

The symptoms of retroperitoneal fibrosis can include backache, fatigue, weight loss, low-grade fever, difficulty passing urine and leg pain and swelling.

Retroperitoneal fibrosis is diagnosed with an investigative test called an 'intravenous pyelogram' (IVP). If fibrosis is present in the abdomen, this test will show an obstruction of one or both of the tubes (ureters) leading from the kidneys to the bladder. Other investigative tests may also be used where appropriate.

Since fibrosis can also form in the chest cavity, a chest X-ray or other imaging will be done if there is difficulty breathing or tightness and pain in the chest, which would indicate possible fibrosis around the lungs and heart structures.

Another type of antiserotonin agent is called pizotifen. Although it is not generally as effective as methysergide, it is usually better tolerated and does not have the potential to cause retroperitoneal fibrosis. In studies, one-third to one-half of the participants improved while taking pizotifen. Weight gain and drowsiness are common side effects.

Anticonvulsants

Certain anticonvulsant or antiseizure medications are sometimes used for migraine prevention, after other therapies have been tried. This medication is, once again, prescribed not because epilepsy is present, but to help with the migraine. Studies have shown that both valproic acid and sodium valproate are effective for migraine prevention. However, they must not be used during pregnancy. As a safety measure, liver function is sometimes monitored periodically through blood tests while someone is taking these medications. An anticonvulsant called gabapentin has been used successfully in a few patients with migraine and facial pain. Topiramate has been shown to help sometimes in migraine and in cluster. Studies are underway with gabapentin and topiramate.

Antihistamines

Non-prescription antihistamines are not used for migraine prevention. The anti-serotonin properties of a particular medication called cyproheptadine may make it a useful migraine preventive but there are no published studies. It is not usually very effective in adults, but it may help some children. It works along the serotonin pathway and also seems to prevent blood vessels from constricting or dilating. It can cause sleepiness, so it is usually taken at bedtime. It can also cause weight gain, like most migraine preventives.

Clonidine

Clonidine is a medication that some doctors prescribe with varying success for migraine prevention. Clonidine stabilizes blood vessels throughout the body by preventing them from overdistending or from narrowing too much. However, clinical-trial results using clonidine have been mixed. Overall results of clonidine's ability to prevent migraine attacks are quite poor, so it is not often used.

Long-acting opioids

There is much controversy regarding the use of these long-acting narcotic preparations for the prevention of very stubborn, severe daily headache disorders that are not reduced by any other means. These long-acting opioids include methadone, fentanyl and sustained-release morphine sulfate (a long-acting form of morphine). The safety and effectiveness of this form of treatment have not been determined and it is only very rarely used as a last-resort form of headache prevention.

Taking your preventive medicines

It is considered useful to continue taking preventive medications when the frequency of attacks experienced is reduced by half. Since breakthrough attacks are likely to occur, sufferers on a prophylactic regime should speak to their doctor about how to manage any remaining attacks. It is always important to report any side effects directly to the doctor and an effort should be made not to miss doses of the prophylactic medication. The medication should be taken at the same time each day, whenever possible. Consult your chemist about possible drug interactions.

Preventive medications must be taken every day whether there is a headache present or not. They will not be helpful if taken only when an attack strikes. Stay in touch with the doctor so that necessary adjustments may be made to the ongoing treatment and never share medications with friends or family members.

Botulinum toxin injections

Recent research has focused interest on a yet-to-be-approved use of botulinum toxin type A for the prevention of migraine and chronic tension-type headache. Although additional research is still needed, botulinum toxin type A injections every three to four months may reduce the need for daily acute or preventive medication.

Botulinum toxin type A is a protein structure produced by bacteria that can cause botulism (a type of food poisoning). In small doses, it is currently being used safely to treat many conditions from wrinkles and crossed eyes to cerebral palsy.

Why these injections appear to work for people with headache isn't fully understood, but most researchers believe that the injections decrease muscle tone by reducing the release of the neurochemical acetylcholine. But since other brain chemicals that could be more centrally related to migraine may also be reduced by these injections, there is speculation that there may be more to the mechanism than simply relaxing sore, overworked muscles.

To date, botulinum toxin injections have most often been given to headache patients via symmetrical injections into certain muscles – predominantly in the forehead and temples. No serious adverse events have been reported, and drooping of the upper eyelids, lasting a week or two, has been the most commonly reported significant side effect. There may be temporary pain at the injection site. It is expected that such effects will happen less as we gain more experience and knowledge regarding optimal dosing and injection sites.

Studies are currently under way to determine the best dose, best site(s) of injection and which type of headache and/or headache sufferers benefit most. However, botulinum toxin injections are expensive.

The emergency treatment of migraine

A 1990 study showed that 14 per cent of migraine sufferers attend an emergency department at one time or another for treatment of a severe or unremitting attack. Some migraine attacks will simply not respond to the treatments available outside the hospital. If vomiting is present, migraine patients can become dehydrated and administration of intravenous fluids may be necessary.

All headache sufferers should proceed immediately to the emergency department if any of the following signs of possible life-threatening problems exist:

- first episode of the worst headache ever experienced (particularly if it came on suddenly)
- severe headache that comes on suddenly with physical exertion (including sexual activity)
- headache associated with other unusual symptoms such as limb weakness
- loss of consciousness with the headache
- headache associated with a stiff neck
- headache associated with a fever
- new headache or change in usual headache after age 50
- headache associated with visual problems (other than the temporary visual disorder of migraine with aura).

In addition, people who experience any other unusual symptoms or change in the quality, character, location or frequency of their usual migraine should check with their doctor without delay.

If you are caught in the jaws of a prolonged migraine attack, your decision to attend the emergency department will probably be made after you've tried every medication in your cabinet, in addition to every non-drug strategy known to man (including prayer and bargaining with the powers that be). The car, taxi or bus trip was probably a brutal endurance test. Now it's time to face the unfamiliar ground of an emergency department.

Most people hate hospitals at the best of times. When your head is throbbing, you're close to vomiting and the light feels like blades piercing your eyes, you're not in any mood to handle the waiting room at emergency. The bad news is that you must. Despite the bright lights, sounds, commotion and sometimes foul smell of the hospital, treatment for your migraine begins with explaining yourself and registering at the front desk.

Upon arrival at most emergency departments, you will first encounter a triage nurse. The nurse will probably ask a series of questions about your head pain and other symptoms. The information gathered helps the nurse to assess the urgency of your medical needs. This assessment of urgency can anger even the most patient migraine sufferer. When you decided to come to the hospital, you did so because you found yourself in a terrible predicament. No matter what you did, your head pain and other symptoms just wouldn't stop. Now that you're finally there, you want relief fast. The trouble is, the staff must attend to patients with *life-threatening* needs first: people with heart attacks, strokes, suicidal thoughts, haemorrhages and other problems that simply can't wait. And although it is torture to be kept waiting, your life is not threatened. Try to make the best of it. Ask if there is anywhere less bright and noisy to wait. Since lying flat will probably make your head pain worse, sitting in a chair or on a stretcher with your head raised at least 45 degrees may be preferable. A basin can be provided by the staff if nausea or vomiting is part of your attack.

When the doctor arrives to speak with you, he or she will have to perform a neurological evaluation. People who have suffered severe migraine attacks for years and know that this attack is definitely a migraine, and is just like the other bad ones, often can't understand why they have to be 'poked and prodded' by the doctor. There are two reasons the doctor must examine you. The first is to rule out other (potentially life-threatening) causes of your symptoms. Although ominous causes of head pain are only rarely detected, they occur often enough to warrant thorough investigation of each and every migraine sufferer each and every time he or she attends the emergency department. The second reason is to ensure that there are no other health problems present that would preclude the use of any medications. Be sure to tell the doctor of any allergies or coexisting health problems.

Some migraine sufferers have attempted to bypass the neurological examination and 'question period' in the emergency department by having the doctor who usually treats their migraine provide them with a note to hand to the emergency staff. Usually these notes contain confirmation that the patient gets migraine and recommendations on which medications to use to stop the attack. But there is no guarantee, for either the migraine sufferer or the emergency-room doctor, that another problem hasn't developed since the note was written. In addition, emergency-room doctors are not likely to abandon their own judgement and recommendations for treatment. So although such notes may be a helpful way for your usual doctor to communicate with emergency staff, an examination will still be carried out and a treatment plan will be developed.

Until recently, the treatment of choice among emergency departments for unremitting migraine pain involved the administration of narcotics, usually in the form of an injection given into the hip or through an intravenous drip. Narcotics such as pethidine are no longer usually considered the treatment of choice for migraine – unless there are reasons why other medications can't be used – for several reasons. First, the type of migraine attack that sends sufferers to the emergency department most often is called 'status migrainosus'. This unremitting headache may be driven by a vicious pain cycle involving the use of painkillers. No matter how many painkillers you take, the attack cycle just can't be broken. Adding another painkiller onto the pile may bring temporary relief, but it will ultimately contribute to the problem of rebound headache once its effects wear off. The relief experienced from the narcotic will probably wear off just as you get home, and you may find yourself having to head back to emergency before long.

The movement toward not using narcotics to treat migraine necessitated a search for effective alternatives. It's fine to say something isn't good because its effects are only temporary, but the medical profession had to come up with something to replace narcotics. A variety of non-narcotic preparations have been shown to be as effective as narcotics, or more so. They can break status migrainosus and the vicious cycle of rebound headache.

In the hospital setting, migraine sufferers can often avail themselves of non-narcotic treatments not usually available in a doctor's office. If vomiting has been present for an extended period of time, dehydration may result, and it may not be possible to get down or keep down oral medications.

Fluids may be given intravenously in this situation.

Medications sometimes used in the emergency department, given intravenously or by injection, for the treatment of migraine include:

- migraine-specific treatment such as DHE, often with an antinausea preparation
- antinausea preparations such as domperidone or metoclopramide
- injectable non-steroidal anti-inflammatories such as ketorolac
- steroids (not the body-building type)
- antinausea/antipsychotics (dopamine antagonists) that have pain-relieving properties and may have direct anti-migraine properties, such as prochlorperazine or chlorpromazine
- intravenous magnesium sulphate.

Sumatriptan injections are sometimes used in the emergency department, but since migraine sufferers can administer sumatriptan with the auto-injecting syringe, the trip to the emergency department to obtain it is usually not necessary.

The shift to avoiding the use of narcotics for the treatment of migraine has a further benefit to migraine sufferers. In the past, migraine sufferers who arrived at the emergency department in the throes of an attack were often labelled 'drug addicts'. Suspicious doctors and nurses were apt to interpret a request for a particular narcotic as 'drug-seeking behaviour'. They were not justified in this labelling, but they often came by their attitude honestly. There are drug addicts who pretend to be in pain to get a 'fix'. A staff member who has been tricked before may be suspicious next time around. Nobody says it is right to question a patient's honesty, but it's plain to see why some medical staff would. Doctors and nurses are legally accountable, right down to the last milligram of narcotic they give, so they are bound to be judicious. Since there are no lab tests to prove beyond a doubt that a migraine is in progress, some choose to be suspicious of most migraine sufferers. The new advances that have brought migraine sufferers more effective relief through non-narcotic alternatives are indeed welcome. Even more effective treatments are under development in laboratories around the world.

During the throes of severe attacks, some sufferers experience a level of desperation higher than ever before. Some can even be driven to contemplate suicide. Indeed, migraine may coexist in people suffering major depression. One study showed a higher incidence of suicide and thoughts of suicide in people who have migraine with aura, and migraine with aura coupled with major depression, than in people who do not suffer from either disorder. Those who experience thoughts of suicide should go or be taken to the emergency department immediately. Migraine and major depression are both treatable medical disorders. There is help and hope available 24 hours a day at the emergency department.

The emergency department staff are available to address urgent needs for headache treatment, but the family doctor (sometimes in consultation with a neurologist) is very often the person to consult to develop and modify an ongoing migraine treatment plan. Usual migraine treatment is best done outside of the emergency department, with healthcare practitioners who are familiar with your individual case history.

Enlisting your doctor's help

Many migraine sufferers report instances in which they have
been left feeling as though their migraine is not being taken
seriously enough by healthcare practitioners. When they are
told that their pain is not real or that they are bringing it
upon themselves, a great deal of needless emotional grief is
caused. You know that your suffering is very real and that
you need the help of a qualified practitioner to gain control
over it.

Most migraine sufferers start by enlisting the help of their
family doctor or general practitioner. Sometimes, but not
always, the doctor will refer you to a consulting neurologist to confirm an initial diagnosis, or later on, if the
migraine is resistant to the treatment the doctor prescribed.
Neurologists are very familiar with migraine, but a referral
from the doctor is usually needed to secure a neurology
appointment.

The neurologist's role is usually to act as a consultant.
Neurologists do not tend to monitor their migraine patients
over extended periods as a matter of practice; rather, they
consult, providing an opinion in diagnosis, and are often
asked to recommend treatment plans. Often the neurologist
will see the migraine patient, prescribe treatment and send
a referral note to the family doctor. The neurologist will give
instructions to the patient (and sometimes to the doctor)
regarding follow-up. If the medications or other treatments
are ineffective, stop working, or cause side effects, consult
the doctor. If the treatment was prescribed by a neurologist,
many migraine sufferers think that that particular prescription was the best or only treatment available and there is
nothing left for them to try if it doesn't work. The neurologist has prescribed what he or she feels is the best treatment

to try first, based on the patient's symptoms and profile, and the doctor's past experience. But it certainly isn't the only option available. If the first, second or even third plan fails, it is important to keep trying. It is up to patients to keep the doctor informed about their response to therapies, so that the doctor can make adjustments to the medications or treatments. So when accepting a prescription from a neurologist, ask whom to see regarding future fine-tuning of the treatment. Some neurologists prefer that their patients call their offices directly for follow-up appointments; others prefer that their patients see the family doctor, who can then reach the neurologist by telephone or letter for consultation.

Depending on where you live, you may be referred to a headache clinic. In the UK, most headache patients are seen in neurology clinics, although there are a growing number of specialist headache clinics.

You must participate in your own treatment, starting with minimizing your exposure to triggers, getting regular exercise balanced with adequate rest, looking at your psychological health and discontinuing any daily, or almost daily, use of any amount of any type of painkiller.

When you arrive for your appointment at either the family doctor's or the specialist's office, open up the lines of communication. Be clear and concise about your symptoms, and make notes beforehand if it helps (see Chapter 2 for a list of questions to ponder before the appointment). There is no lab test for migraine, and your doctor can't tell from the outside how bad the pain is, how it affects your life and what all your symptoms are. Be honest about how you currently treat your headaches. If you have found yourself in the cycle of taking medication daily, tell your doctor how much you actually take – the doctor is there to help you break the cycle of rebound headache if you find yourself in it. Ask questions, and listen closely to what the doctor says. Talk about treatments with and without medications, and what to expect from any prescribed treatment, such as potential side effects; how much and how often to take any medications; whom your next appointment should be with; and how soon you need to see a doctor again.

On your return visits, or before if necessary, be sure to keep the doctor informed about the success of your treatment so that any necessary adjustments can be made. And always report any side effects experienced without delay. If the first treatment doesn't work, see your doctor again. There are many, many treatment options available and most people try several before they find what works best for them.

What should you expect from your relationship with your doctor? You should expect to be met with compassionate concern. You deserve to be listened to. Your doctor should become your partner in overcoming migraine and should be open to examining your triggers, exercise pattern or psychological situation in an effort to manage your migraine. If you get the impression that you are expected to do what the doctor says without discussion or question, that isn't much of a partnership. You must receive adequate explanation about your therapy, and you must take an active role in decision making.

11
Comfort Measures and Home Remedies

Your doctor has helped you with medication; you've set up routines for sleeping, eating and exercise; and you've tried to avoid your usual triggers. But unfortunately there is no cure, and the best-laid plans cannot keep migraine from occasionally rearing its ugly head.

When an attack comes, make certain that those close to you understand your need for special attention. Rally your friends and family to take any responsibilities off your hands for a few hours and ask them to be nearby in case the attack is severe.

Often migraine sufferers ignore the symptoms of an impending attack. Research indicates that, hours before an attack begins, your stomach stops working properly and becomes less able to absorb drugs. So, if medication has been prescribed by your doctor to ease the attack, make sure to take it as soon as you are certain that a migraine is setting in.

Over time, many migraine sufferers find effective ways to

either stave off a full-blown attack, reduce its severity or simply add a measure of comfort. Over the years, many people have shared with me some of their favourite tricks. Coupled with my own experience and the advice my mother once gave me, here are some tips to ponder. Although many of them are not explained by our current scientific knowledge, you may find them worth trying.

When an attack strikes, find a dark, quiet room in which to lie down. Use a pillow to elevate your head, as lying flat will make the throbbing worse. Change into comfortable clothing if you are at home (flannel pyjamas or nightdresses are great). Sleep is still the best way to get through an attack. Many will wake to find the migraine has disappeared. In the meantime, you may find a gel cold pack or cold facecloth will comfort your temples, forehead or the back of your neck. Cold water can be splashed on the face for relief no matter where you are. A bag of frozen peas (reusable, but don't eat the peas) or a balloon filled with cold water and tied off may work just fine. While cold is often good for the head, some prefer heat. Others find it helpful to apply heat or warm water to the hands and feet, as warming them can bring down excess blood from the head. Some sufferers report the ability to stop an attack from progressing by running their hands under cold water, or by holding ice cubes in the palms of their hands at the first sign of an attack.

Lying still will probably make you feel better during an attack. Sudden lurches to the lavatory can be avoided by keeping a bucket and fresh water nearby if vomiting is part of the attack. Some sufferers prefer to stay in the bathroom, and find a warm bath will relax tense muscles and help reduce blood flow to the head. It may even be especially helpful to put a cold pack on your head while in the warm bath. Alternatively, a shower will be comforting to some; the water stream will provide a scalp massage when directed on the head (with or without a pulsating shower head).

Some even find that food or drink helps them. Some sip cold water, some a herbal tea. Some find that the actual action of eating somehow brings temporary relief. A 1993 British study by Dr J.N. Blau asked migraine sufferers what they could eat or drink during their attacks. Of the 109 sufferers surveyed, 59 could not take any food and 50 said they could eat during an attack. Of the 50 participants who could eat, 38 ate dry carbohydrate foods; 5 ate small amounts of their regular diet; 4 ate normally; and 3 ate lighter foods.

Sufferers who don't find caffeine a trigger swear by a strong cup of coffee, which may help by constricting swollen blood vessels and by hastening the emptying of the stomach. Ginger root in warm water or tea, or the ginger in ginger ale or ginger beer, can act as an antinausea remedy.

One sufferer swore by swallowing a tablespoon of honey at the earliest sign of an attack to prevent the migraine from progressing. A caller to a radio programme said the pain of his migraine could be diminished by eating a salty pickle during the early stages. Others swear by chewing gum to prevent attacks from becoming full blown (beware of aspartame in some sugar-free gum as it is a potential trigger for some).

Eye care should be attended to during an attack. Contact-lens wearers often gain added comfort by removing their lenses. Glasses must be substituted if the sufferer is staying up out of bed. Women should remove eye make-up (especially mascara). Commercially available cosmetic eye gels (available at the cosmetic counters in major department stores) can be used to provide a delicate massage of the eye area. Storing the gel in the refrigerator will provide an even more refreshing tonic to the eyes.

Each migraine sufferer is different, so it's important for you to try different safe methods to determine what will help you get through or avoid an attack.

There was an interesting study published in 2000 examining 'Tricks to Relieve Migraine Attacks'. It reported that, with the exception of taking medication, the best tricks for relieving migraine pain were pressing the site of the pain against a hand or a pillow, isolating oneself from sound and light and applying cold to the head. Other comfort measures you can consider including are complementary therapies such as self-hypnosis, biofeedback, yoga, acupuncture or acupressure, or massage. The following chapter looks at some of the options available.

12
Complementary Therapies

If you are thinking of seeing someone other than a medical doctor about your migraine, you may be about to join the growing crowd of people who are seeking to supplement their standard medical care with safe complementary therapies.

Not so long ago, the medical community tended to dismiss so-called alternatives, largely because of the lack of scientific evidence supporting the safety and effectiveness of the therapies. Today we are beginning to see a blending of modern medicine with ancient medicine as clinical trials, detailed case studies and good investigation and safety standards are being developed for complementary medicine. Although there are a growing number of safe, complementary practices available to headache sufferers and guidelines for the non-drug management of migraine have been published by experts, most of the therapies mentioned in this chapter have not been proved by properly designed clinical trials to be safe and effective. Always consult your doctor before embarking on any therapy.

Finding an alternative practitioner: how to spot a quack

Complementary medicine is not as well regulated as conventional medicine, and there are some less than ethical practitioners out there. Here are some tips and hints on determining whether your complementary treatment is valid and safe.

Think twice about seeing a therapist who will not allow you to see anyone else at the same time. Always see a medical doctor for the initial diagnosis, and follow up continuously to have your progress monitored. Always return to your medical doctor if there is a change in your symptoms and before you embark on any new therapy. Ethical and safe complementary practitioners should be willing to work with your medical doctor.

If the product or therapy cannot be supported by valid research, think twice. Testimonials from the manufacturer or one or two people are not enough. And if the therapy seems excessive, requiring large doses, multiple potions and supplements, office visits three times a week for ten years or a second mortgage on your home to pay for it, watch out.

If the therapist says, 'Doctors don't like me because *I* have the cure,' don't believe it. If the therapist claims to be able to cure you completely with a magic answer, he or she is not telling the truth. Ask the therapist if you can speak to other clients with migraine he or she has treated, to discuss their experience. And finally, if it doesn't feel right, don't do it.

If any of the options described in this book or others you may come across sound interesting to you, make an appointment for consultation with a practitioner in your area. Use the phone directory, look in the paper and ask around to find those nearby. Ask the practitioner about qualifications and whether his or her area of speciality is regulated by a professional organization. Look in the phone book to see if there are professional associations for the type of therapist you are looking for in your area and call to see if they can recommend qualified practitioners or tell you what to watch for. Good therapists will take the time to explain the therapy or treatment to you before you make any type of commitment. They should allow you time to examine the way you feel about the treatment, to ask any questions and to talk it over with your medical doctor.

The placebo effect

'Placebo' is defined in *The Oxford Paperback Dictionary* as 'a harmless substance given as if it were medicine, to humour a patient or as a dummy pill etc. in a controlled experiment'. Perhaps it is the notion that placebos may be given simply 'to humour a patient' that makes most people uncomfortable with the idea of them and their ability to subconsciously 'trick' patients into feeling better. But placebos and the placebo effect are scientifically valid and should be taken seriously.

Let's look, first, at the use of placebos in controlled experiments. When studying the effects of new medications, researchers compare the ability of the medication to alleviate symptoms with the ability of a placebo to alleviate symptoms. Good studies are 'double-blinded', that is, neither the patient nor the healthcare provider knows whether the active drug or a placebo is being administered. The study medication is packaged in the lab by a third person, who numbers the medication and keeps the code that will identify which patient received what substance when the research results are tabulated. It is important to use placebos in research. If the medication is shown to have effect in comparison with the results obtained in patients treated with placebos, it becomes possible to prove without a doubt that the success of the medication was true. Without the direct comparison, sceptics would argue that perhaps the condition cleared up on its own. They might also say that the patient simply felt better as a result of the tender loving concern received.

In headache studies, the percentage of those experiencing the placebo effect (the improvement of patients that occurs after they receive a placebo) is higher than in studies of many other disorders. This should not be interpreted as an indication that headache sufferers 'put on' their symptoms. The success of placebos is probably a result of the brain's higher power to heal itself through suggestion. In giving a placebo, the researchers are not fooling the patients; rather, they are fooling the neurobiochemical functions of the brain. The end result is a release by the brain of chemicals that make the pain subside. This 'placebo effect' is not strong enough to warrant withholding active treatment in favour of sugar pills as common practice, but the 'mind over matter' principle is believed by many doctors and researchers to be behind the effectiveness of many complementary therapies. The subconscious mind *can* be influenced to heal through the power of suggestion.

In drug research, the patient and doctor can be 'blinded' to what is the active drug and what is a placebo simply by making the placebo pills or injections look exactly the same as the 'real stuff' in colour, shape, design and packaging. In most complementary therapies, however, it is not possible to use the double-blind. Take, for instance, acupuncture. The patient knows whether or not the needles are going in, and the acupuncturist knows whether or not he or she is using the technique. Therefore, the placebo effect cannot be measured in the study of most complementary therapies, rendering any results obtained 'non-scientific' in the opinion of many experts. But just because we don't know how the relief was obtained (whether it was a result of the treatment or a result of the brain's subconscious reaction) doesn't mean that the relief wasn't real or valuable. In other words, if it works safely, it has value. If it works through tricking the brain into releasing pain-relieving chemicals, it is valuable, even if it is a placebo.

Biofeedback

Biofeedback has been shown to be useful in reducing both the severity and the frequency of attacks for some headache and migraine sufferers. How it works is not completely understood, and the placebo effect may be involved. Biofeedback takes discipline to master, and it is not effective for everyone. As with most new things, children often pick up the new skill faster than adults, but, with determination, adults can become just as good at it, usually within four to six weeks. And although reaching for medication may bring faster results, biofeedback brings long-lasting results with almost no risk of negative side effects. It can be useful on its own, or in combination with medication to enhance the effects of the medicine and, possibly, to reduce the amount of medicine needed. Biofeedback training can involve a substantial investment of time, and even money in some regions, but it is eventually possible to learn to practise biofeedback techniques anywhere and anytime.

Biofeedback is taught by trained therapists. The psychology

or psychiatry departments of large hospitals often teach biofeedback, as do many independent therapists. Listings of biofeedback therapists near you can sometimes be found in the Yellow Pages under 'biofeedback', 'stress management', or 'personal counselling'. Your family doctor may also know of biofeedback practitioners in the area.

The biofeedback therapist works with the migraine sufferer through several sessions. The aim is to learn how to control subconscious processes within the body. Body awareness and breathing exercises, progressive relaxation, guided imagery, hand warming and self-directed phrases to encourage relaxation are the types of techniques often taught. You will initially learn biofeedback using a computer. Electromyographic monitors (also known as EMG monitors) use adhesive patches that are applied to the forehead to monitor muscle contraction. Another type of biofeedback monitor measures your finger temperature through a thermistor, an adhesive pad that is applied to the finger. Types of biofeedback include thermal biofeedback, EMG biofeedback, cephalic vasomotor biofeedback and autogenic training.

So, what does mastering biofeedback lead to? For most, a decrease in the number of headaches and a reduction in their severity. But biofeedback also leads to an elevation in mood, a better night's sleep and an increased sense of power and control. If you are considering experimenting in the areas of meditation, massage or other alternative approaches, biofeedback may be a good first step. It is one of the few complementary treatments for migraine that has been carefully studied and reported on.

Hypnotherapy

Although stress is not a *cause* of migraine, for some people it may be a triggering factor. In learning to gain the upper hand over stress, many migraine sufferers find hypnotherapy and self-hypnosis to be helpful. These techniques are also useful in dealing with the pain of migraine when an attack occurs.

Hypnosis does not take over your mind, cause you to lose control or make you say or do unusual things. Hypnosis is a very deep form of relaxation – close to how you feel when you are about to fall asleep. And you can break out of it any time you wish.

Self-hypnosis is the goal in hypnotherapy training. It takes only about half an hour to learn the basics of self-hypnosis, but follow-up sessions are necessary for practice and re-inforcement. Mental attitude is very important, and there will be times early on when you find it difficult to believe that what is being taught can actually work – hence, the need for continuing support from the therapist. Classes should not go on too long, as the goal is self-sufficiency.

Different practitioners employ different techniques in training their patients. Some physicians have special training in clinical hypnosis. Migraine is extremely complex and its treatment demands specialized knowledge and insight.

Most people who have trained themselves in self-hypnosis have experienced some degree of relief. Virtually all have found it refreshing, relaxing and interesting, and some have carried on to experiment with its use in other areas of their lives.

Meditation

The Maharishi Mahesh Yogi taught the Beatles a technique known as 'transcendental meditation', or TM. Many other people have now caught on to India's approach to reducing stress and expanding good health and awareness by inducing a state of extreme relaxation with increased wakefulness.

Yogis give instruction on how to bring about a refreshing state of mind. The meditator sits with eyes closed and focuses all thoughts and awareness inward. TM may assist in the release of beneficial body chemicals, reducing blood pressure and improving cell metabolism. TM can be practised anywhere and should be practised regularly for best results.

Relaxation

There are many commercially available relaxation tapes, CDs and videos. Some are designed specifically to assist migraine or headache sufferers. These guide the listener through breathing exercises and progressive relaxation and help in imagining pleasant circumstances through guided imagery. They are often designed to help the listener access information about the generation of negative thoughts and feelings, and they use specifically targeted phrases and auditory images. Relaxation tapes and other aids are often found for sale in bookstores and healthfood stores, or they may be borrowed from libraries. Never listen to one in the car. It is best to sit in a comfortable chair or to lie down on a bed or sofa in a quiet place while absorbing their relaxing effects.

When you are in pain, exercising the imagination can be helpful. Some imagine themselves on a paradise island. Some recall very pleasant events or situations, or occupy their

Stress busters

Migraine sufferers must be careful to minimize any harmful effects stress may have as a potential trigger of their attacks. Stress is present in everyone's life. These simple stress-busting strategies may help you manage stress and build a healthier lifestyle:

- get plenty of rest

- participate in an aerobic activity (even brisk walking is good) for twenty to thirty minutes, three or four times every week

- eat sensible, regular meals, and consume only those foods that are trigger-free for you

- communicate your problems, concerns and thoughts – don't 'bottle them up'

- identify sources of stress in your life and make a promise to yourself to begin working to improve problem areas

- learn how to 'do nothing' on occasion: if you sit down on the couch to relax, don't pick up the phone, a magazine and the television remote control all at the same time.

thoughts with counting or repeating pleasant-sounding words (like 'soft') in order to avoid focusing on the pain. Controlled breathing exercises can be helpful in many painful or stressful situations. Breathing in pain relief and breathing out pain, or breathing in imagined fresh, pastel colours (so-called good colours) while exhaling dark colours (bad colours), are useful exercises.

Massage

Recently, therapeutic massage has become popular. Massage therapy involves the manipulation of the soft tissues of the body (skin, muscles and the structures contained in them) for therapeutic effect. Massage therapy is believed to create a feeling of well-being through assisting blood flow. Massage can relieve pressure and tension that have accumulated in large muscle groups (usually the neck and upper body in headache sufferers).

Massage therapy is offered by registered massage therapists. Migraine sufferers interested in trying massage therapy should seek out a fully qualified professional. Massage therapists complete many hours of training at approved schools of massage, and they must pass rigorous examinations. Therapy is individually designed and may vary in duration from 30 to 90 minutes. It may include Swedish massage, paraffin wax treatments, hydrotherapy, cryotherapy, deep-tissue massage or others. Prices vary from therapist to therapist, depending on what components of therapy are involved.

Courses on massage techniques are available. Check with community schools and massage clinics near you. Many sufferers report that taking a massage course with their partner is fun, in addition to being helpful and healthful for both the migraine sufferer and the partner.

Chiropractic treatment

Chiropractors put a different emphasis on why headaches occur and they differ from medical doctors in how they treat migraine. Both groups acknowledge that many factors influence migraine, including inherited susceptibility, the blood vessels surrounding the brain, brain chemistry and the environment and general psychological health. However, chiropractors often disagree with doctors when it comes to the source of the pain, the diagnosis of the different types of headache and the treatment of the pain.

Chiropractors believe that all headaches not caused by sinister conditions such as tumours or haemorrhages are caused by spinal misalignments, abnormal biomechanics and other special imbalances that lead to subluxation (spinal misalignment). They believe the spinal misalignment, in turn, leads to abnormal functioning of the nervous system, muscles, joints and internal organs, thereby leading to headaches. Chiropractors believe the spinal problems actually cause the whole problem of headache and that there is no causative difference between tension-type headaches and migraine.

Chiropractors use diverse treatments to correct the spinal imbalances, including hands-on techniques to manipulate and adjust the spinal vertebrae. These techniques are designed to restore normal functioning, correct the causes of irritation to the nervous system, increase the range of motion and (according to chiropractic theory) correct the underlying cause of the pain. Many holistic chiropractors also employ techniques such as nutritional counselling, relaxation training, exercise therapy and body-mechanics education.

One of the difficulties in assessing the effectiveness of chiropractic treatment for headache is the non-scientific design of many of the studies that have been done. However, one controlled study performed in Australia in 1976 apparently showed that chiropractic adjustment provided an effective treatment for migraine. But, like many other treatments for migraine, it is not 100 per cent effective, and it does carry with it the potential for serious side effects, which must be discussed with qualified practitioners before going ahead. Stroke, although rare, is the most serious possible complication of neck manipulation. Chiropractic treatment will not be chosen as a treatment for all, but it can be a helpful part of migraine management.

Transcutaneous electrical nerve stimulation

Transcutaneous electrical nerve stimulation (TENS) involves the application of stick-on electrode pads (usually on the forehead, temples and upper back/shoulder area when treating headache) which are attached by wires to a unit emitting high-frequency, low-intensity electrical stimulation. The exact mechanism behind TENS is unknown, but some people believe it works on the gate-control theory of pain. Researchers think that there is a 'gate' that controls the amount of pain we feel. This gate can be closed by overriding its ability to let pain in with another non-painful message or stimulus (in other words, if the entrance is blocked with one impulse, the painful one can't get through). The principle of the gate-control theory is what makes rubbing your elbow feel better when you bang it on the edge of the table.

Studies have shown TENS to be of help to about 50 per cent of those who suffer from chronic pain. Although it hasn't been studied extensively for use in headache, research suggests it may be helpful for some as a supplemental therapy.

Herbal remedies

Our earliest ancestors knew a great deal about herbal remedies and their healing power. Indeed, 25 per cent of modern prescription drugs are derived from plants. However, compared with today's medicines, relatively little scientific research has been done to support the effectiveness or safety of many herbal therapies. It is extremely costly to conduct the research needed to obtain approval of a new drug. Manufacturers of drugs can patent new medications to protect their investment, but herbal researchers can't patent a plant.

One of the most popular herbal therapies for the prevention of migraine attacks is feverfew, or *Tanacetum parthenium*. Feverfew is a plant from the chrysanthemum family whose leaves have been eaten by migraine sufferers in Britain to prevent attacks for almost two decades. A scientific study of feverfew was published in the *Lancet* in 1988. The study of 72 people showed that two months of treatment with feverfew was associated with a reduction in the mean number and severity of attacks, as well as in the degree of vomiting. There were no serious side effects reported in this study. One must be cautioned against basing individual therapy on the results of a single study, however, because a 1998 review of all published feverfew trials concluded that 'the clinical effectiveness of feverfew in the prevention of migraine has not been established beyond reasonable doubt.'

Feverfew is intended for use as a preventive therapy. This means it should be taken every day, whether there is a headache or not. It isn't likely to be effective if only taken for relief of attacks in progress.

The active ingredient in feverfew is thought to be parthenolide. The amount of parthenolide present in commercially available products varies widely and some brands of feverfew have been found to contain no active ingredient at all!

Feverfew is not suitable for all and can cause mouth or throat ulcers. Other adverse reactions include loss of taste or a bitter taste from chewing the leaves, swelling of the lips, dermatitis, temporary increase in heart rate, abdominal pain or heartburn, dizziness or light-headedness and increased menstrual flow. If use of feverfew is stopped abruptly, about 10 per cent of people experience nervous anxiety, insomnia and muscle and joint stiffness. Severe headaches and nausea may also be components of 'post-feverfew syndrome'. Feverfew's active ingredient also has an effect on blood platelets, so it is important to check with your doctor before starting any treatment with it. It should not be used in pregnancy. Feverfew has still not been fully evaluated for safety and a high degree of responsibility must be exercised when taking this preparation.

Over the years, many other herbal compounds and tonics have been suggested for migraine. Herbal teas and medicines contain active compounds, and it is possible for side effects to occur. For example, the Genesis Research Foundation reported on a study published in *Annals of Internal Medicine* that showed that hepatitis may be caused by herbal preparations containing valerian, asafetida, hops, skullcap, gentian, senna fruit extracts, Chinese herbs, mistletoe and chaparral leaf. Also, germander, a herb commonly used to lose weight, occasionally may cause hepatitis. Fortunately, after use of these herbs was discontinued, the symptoms of hepatitis disappeared, but full recovery took up to six months.

It is best to confer with your doctor and to research what herbal remedies may work safely for you. Find out as much as you can about the product, preparation and person recommending it before you start therapy.

Vitamins, minerals and oils

Vitamin B_2, or riboflavin, has been shown to help prevent migraines when taken daily. In one three-month study, participants who took a high dose of the vitamin (400 milligram) experienced 37 per cent fewer migraines than those who took a placebo. It is thought that the vitamin increases the energy potential of mitochondria, the cells' main source of energy. Studies have shown that migraine sufferers' brains have reduced energy reserves between attacks. A common side effect of high-dose riboflavin is bright yellow urine.

Magnesium has also undergone scientific investigation for use in migraine. In Italy, a small study in which women took a supplement of 360 milligrams of magnesium daily from the fifteenth day of the menstrual cycle until the start of the menstrual period revealed the ability of magnesium to reduce the number of days spent with a migraine. The supplement also reduced some premenstrual symptoms. These findings suggest a possible link between magnesium deficiency and migraine in women. Intravenous magnesium is sometimes given to treat an attack in progress. Dietary sources of magnesium include beans, brown rice and brussels sprouts, as well as sunflower, sesame and pumpkin seeds.

Oils that have varying degrees of success with migraine include omega-3 fish oil and evening primrose oil. It should always be remembered, however, that a person's individual response to *any* treatment or therapy must be considered. For instance, evening primrose oil can actually *cause* headaches for some, and some manufacturers warn that it may trigger migraine in those sufferers whose migraines are alcohol-sensitive.

Homeopathy

Homeopathy is not naturopathy, herbalism or home remedies. It uses medicines on the principle that a substance that produces symptoms in a healthy person cures those symptoms in a sick person. Homeopathy is intended to stimulate the body's natural healing response.

Homeopathic medicines are prepared dilutions of substances.

They are generally made of herbs. Homeopathic practitioners (homeopathists) treat a variety of illnesses, ranging from mild colds to pneumonia. There are no well-conducted, controlled clinical trials to prove or dispute the safety and effectiveness of homeopathic treatment of migraine. However, the International Headache Society's interest in the area has recently prompted the start of the first well-designed study.

If considering homeopathy, you should speak to your own doctor about obtaining a referral. Homeopathy is a complex and difficult subject, requiring years of supervised study and intricate knowledge of the human body. Although homeopathic medicines are derived from natural sources, they still contain active ingredients and are capable of producing side effects, allergic reactions and untoward effects. 'Natural' does not always mean safe, and homeopathic medicines should be approached with the same caution that would be applied to traditional prescription medications.

Yoga

Yoga may be described as a way of life rather than an actual therapy. Yoga is taught by qualified instructors, or yogis. In choosing a yogi, it is imperative to choose someone who has an understanding of migraine in order to design a programme which will help, not worsen, migraine.

Hatha yoga is taught in the western world and is said to control the physical aspects of the body. Certain postures, or *asanas*, are taught and practised to bring awareness and relaxation. It is often practised as a preparation for raja yoga, which is purported to bring mastery of the mind.

Four other yoga paths are intended to bring wisdom, to

practice devotion and worship, to influence consciousness through repeating certain sacred syllables called *mantras*, and to promote the yoga of selfless action and service without thought of oneself, which is called karma yoga.

Yoga requires dedication and a qualified teacher, but the efforts often lead to a more relaxed body and mind. Participants practise the techniques of sitting or lying still in the *asanas*, controlled breathing, thought focusing and meditation. The postures of yoga should not be practised on a full stomach, and many should not be done during pregnancy or within two months after childbirth. Never strain to achieve extreme postures. Always check with a doctor before starting a yoga class, particularly if high or low blood pressure, heart disease, slipped discs, hernias, or back problems are present, or if you have had a recent serious operation.

Acupuncture, acupressure and shiatsu

Acupuncture was developed in China many years ago. Taoist philosophers say that illness occurs when *ch'i*, or life's energy, is out of balance. They believe that 12 energy channels, known as 'meridians', run throughout the body and connect the major bodily organs. The acupuncturist attempts to restore balance between the *yin* (female) and *yang* (male) forces in the body by accessing some of the 800 or so acupuncture points along the meridians. This may be done through the use of extremely fine acupuncture needles of varying lengths. The acupuncturist may alternatively use a soft laser, acupressure, or heat to access the acupuncture points. When acupuncture needles are used, the insertion of these fine needles is so quick and sure that almost no pain is felt. The needles may be left in place for 20 minutes or longer. The acupuncture point may be stimulated by twirling the needle in place. In many cases an electric stimulator is used instead of hand manipulation.

Treatment may be based on assessing pulses at that session and will probably vary from session to session. Many Westerners are surprised to learn that the treatment may take place in an area of the body different from where the pain is located. If you are considering acupuncture, discuss it with your doctor and ask for a referral to a practitioner well trained in the technique.

Some people have reported relief from acupuncture; others have found it to be of no help. A very few found that it temporarily aggravated their migraine.

Shiatsu is a variation of acupuncture often involving deep massage. It is sometimes known as 'acumassage'.

Acupressure, on the other hand, is similar to acupuncture, except the skin is not punctured. Acupressure is applied by the fingers, fingernails or needles with a rounded ballpoint-type end. Other battery-operated or electronic devices work on the same principle, but deliver a low-current electrical charge to the meridian. The same cautions applied to acupuncture apply to acupressure as well.

Many migraine sufferers have discovered on their own that, by pressing on their temples during a painful attack, they can temporarily stop the head pain. Although the exact mechanism underlying this practice is unknown, it is commonly reported to work. A study published in *Headache* by N. Vijayan, showed that a simple elastic headband with rubber discs attached over the temples temporarily relieved 87 per cent of headaches experienced by 23 participants in the study. Migraine sufferers have reported using a variety of homemade devices to compress their temples – a simple scarf or bandanna tied around the head is probably the most common. Others prefer to lie with their 'sore side' down on a firm icepack. Other points to try compressing for temporary relief may include the spot at the back of your head where the very top of your neck meets your skull bone, the centre of your forehead just above the level of your eyebrows, the ridge above your eyes just below your eyebrows, and the area between your thumb and first finger on the non-palm side of your hands.

Naturopathy

Naturopathic medicine involves tailoring a programme of diverse techniques and components to an individual person. The naturopathic doctor customizes a treatment plan that may include the use of acupuncture and oriental medicine, homeopathy, hydrotherapy, spinal manipulation, herbalism or botanical medicine, or dietary counselling, among other methods.

13
Allied Forces: Starting a Self-Help Group

A self-help group brings people with a common concern together to share strength, experience and information. A self-help group can be just a few people meeting for tea, or a larger, more formal gathering. Starting or belonging to a self-help group can be enriching. Simply knowing that you are not alone is empowering. Friendships can grow strong between people who understand from personal experience the difficulties migraine sufferers face in day-to-day life.

Finding a self-help group

Migraine sufferers or their family members and friends who are interested in becoming active in a self-help group can start by trying to determine whether a group already exists. Your first calls should be to the Migraine Action Association and to the Migraine Trust. Good places to search for other groups include classified adverts in the newspaper; church, school or community bulletin boards; and community centres and health clinics. If there isn't a migraine self-help group near you, it may be possible to join a group concerned with a related health problem. For instance, there may be a self-help group for chronic pain in your area. Others prefer to join a group dedicated to assisting with lifestyle changes that might help to improve their migraine. The third option is to consider starting a self-help mutual-aid group for migraine sufferers.

If you are considering starting a self-help group, you must educate yourself about the entire self-help movement. This chapter is intended to provide you with only a general idea of what may be involved in starting and maintaining a self-help group. Authoritative reference material is available for study and must be consulted before embarking on the start-up of a self-help group. See 'Further Resources' for help.

Starting a self-help group

There are several ways to approach starting, running and maintaining a self-help group. Here is a thumbnail sketch of one approach that may work for you.

Pulling together a group of people is time-consuming and challenging. The effort must be shared. Join forces with others to form a founding committee. This founding committee of at least two members will begin initial planning sessions and will organize the first few meetings of the new self-help group. Look for people who have the health, time and energy to 'make it happen.'

Unfortunately, good intentions are not enough. If you are not confident that the group has the strength to succeed, postpone the start-up until you are able to find the help you need.

Trying to do everything yourself will be frustrating, and you are likely to run out of steam before the group is on its feet.

The founding committee will need to make some preliminary decisions. It will need to meet on a few occasions before inviting others to attend an actual self-help group meeting. Initial plans for the first meeting will centre around the following tasks:

- finding a place to meet
- deciding on a time to meet
- advertising the meeting
- appointing a telephone contact person for registration and more information
- appointing a meeting leader/joint leaders (facilitators)
- developing an agenda or general format for the first meeting.

Finding a meeting place may be one of the biggest challenges. Private homes are usually too small, and, sadly, it is probably not a good idea to open your home to the public. Citizen's advice bureaux may be able to help you locate a meeting place. Check with local churches, schools and libraries. If you have no other choice, you may have to rent a room and take up a collection from the group (or charge a set fee, although admittance should never be restricted for any reason) to offset the rent. It is important to have an appropriate room for the group: a room that is too large will make people feel as if there was a disappointing turn-out, and a room that is too small will make people feel crowded and uncomfortable. The telephone contact person must keep a close eye on the number of people registering to avoid either situation. Arrange the chairs so all members can see one another. A large circle may work best.

When thinking of a good time to meet, keep in mind that many in the group will be working outside the home. Most meetings will be best attended if held on a weekday evening. Some prefer a Saturday-morning meeting, but these meetings are likely to be poorly attended during good weather. If your group opts for a weekday evening, time it to occur after dinner. On a full stomach, the group's attention will be more focused (and migraines won't be triggered from delayed meals!). Stick to a regular meeting day and time to allow participants to make plans to attend.

The best ways to advertise your self-help group will vary, depending upon your location and available resources. The key, of course, is to obtain free advertising, as the group will simply not have the budget to pay for adverts. In smaller communities, signs posted in public areas will be effective. In larger towns, however, it may be more of a challenge. Your nearest citizen's advice bureau may be a valuable resource. Newspapers will occasionally make room for public-service adverts. Try sending a short press release to your local radio stations with all the details (call the station to find out to whose attention to send it). Notices on bulletin boards at supermarkets, laundrettes, libraries, schools, churches and citizen's advice bureaux will also help. Consider using computer bulletin boards also. Best of all, word of mouth is the least expensive method of advertising. Tell everyone you know what you are doing; chances are they know a migraine sufferer or two who may have an interest in coming to meetings.

Some groups will have a doctor or other healthcare practitioner involved as a founding member. Many professionals see the need for self-help groups and can assist tremendously in getting the group started. Advertising through medical offices can be very effective. Healthcare professionals may be instrumental in guiding the early meetings and may be valuable information sources for the group. It is very important, however, for the group not to lean on the healthcare professional to provide all the guidance. A self-help group is intended to be directed by its members, all of whom share the same disorder. It is not intended to be a professionally run therapy group. Participation from all members is essential. In the same way, the group should not allow itself to be dominated by one person – professional or not. Nevertheless, some members will naturally be more vocal and outgoing than others. Part of the group facilitator's job will be to ensure that 'quieter ones' are given time and space to participate in their own way.

The person appointed as a telephone contact has an important responsibility. Since the group will not have an office, this person must be committed to acting as the group's receptionist and must have the time to accept calls and to give information about the group. It's a good idea to appoint someone with an answering machine, which can take calls when the person isn't home. You could put a message on the machine giving details (date, time, place, directions and parking information) about the forthcoming meeting. Collect the names, telephone numbers and addresses of those interested in the group and those who attend, in order to stay in touch and to inform them of future meetings and events.

A good meeting must have good direction. A group facilitator is a key person in keeping the meeting on track. It is the responsibility of the group facilitator (or co-facilitators) to act as host and to direct the self-help group participants if the conversation wanders or is dominated by one person. The meeting should not become a gripe session. The term 'group facilitator' is used deliberately rather than 'group leader'. The facilitator's role is not to be boss (or bossy); the facilitator acts as a catalyst in bringing the best of the group together constructively. The facilitator must never dominate the conversation. Although a group facilitator may listen to his or her own voice a fair amount at the early meetings, eventually the whole group will participate, and the group facilitator's role will become one of keeping the group focused and constructive. The facilitator must pay close attention and can often be helpful in summarizing discussion, in unconditionally accepting what is being said or in suggesting ways of tackling difficulties. The group facilitator's behaviour will be infectious. A calm, caring, encouraging group facilitator who accepts all members and shows an interest in what they are saying will impart warmth and friendliness and lead a good meeting. Some groups will stay with the same facilitator; others will take turns chairing the meetings (a true self-help group rotates the role of facilitator). The facilitator may also be given meeting-specific tasks (like opening and locking up the room, arranging for refreshments, etc.).

At the early meetings, members of the group will get to know one another. Sharing stories, tips on coping and names of doctors and medications are frequent items for discussion. At later meetings, the group can focus its attention on particular subjects, such as the triggers of migraine, complementary therapies or other migraine-related topics. The group facilitator should try to keep a positive tone, or at least to wind up the meeting on a good note. Although venting criticism, frustration, anger and other feelings will certainly be on the agenda, the focus should be on improving the situation and not on the feelings of helplessness it can create. Self-help group meetings should never be allowed to be destructive.

As time passes, the group will become cohesive and make

some decisions about itself. Rules for behaviour may be set down. The group may decide to orchestrate meetings around a particular format. Some publications suggest a formal agenda for meetings with defined periods to socialize and to air concerns. Participants, be they in a formal or an informal group, will begin to voice their expectations after a time. Since different people may envision the self-help group in different ways, there is bound to be some conflict at this stage. Some people will choose to leave the group. It would be rare if all members found what they were looking for in any single group. There will be natural ups and downs; the founding members should not take the 'downs' personally, and should strive to remain positive and optimistic. It is important for the group to move ahead and adhere to healthy goals of mutual self-help and healing.

Once a group has ironed out the early wrinkles, it can begin to function as a unit. Although disagreements will occur, they are not usually insurmountable. The camaraderie of people united for the same purpose can be very positive. There is much the group can do to bring strength to its participants through self-help. The group can also act to raise awareness of migraine through public activities. Committees can be struck to raise money for group activities, special projects or awareness programmes. Telephone committees can be set up to allow group participants to reach a fellow group member by phone for friendly support. Members of the group must be encouraged to be creative in their approach to mutual self-help. How about inviting family and friends to a 'no red wine or mature cheese' migraine soirée? Activities and actions that foster togetherness and good spirits should be encouraged.

Self-help groups meet on an ongoing basis. Belonging to a group allows a person to take responsibility for his or her own care and to access a network of information and support that is vital to migraine sufferers. Continued participation in the group can be satisfying and worthwhile. For some, however, participation will be sporadic, usually in times of crisis. Others will only come out to one or two meetings a year. That's fine, too. You may see these people from time to time at educational seminars or other events. Keep them informed of the activities of the group. Simply knowing that there is somewhere to turn should they need the group's help is comforting.

Joining, founding, participating in or checking out a self-help group is a practical way to begin to gain control over migraine. Self-help groups help to fill the void of information and support that many migraine sufferers feel exists. However, the information shared in a self-help group should never become a substitute for medical care.

14
A Quick Reference: Short Answers to Frequently Asked Questions

Q: What causes migraine?
A: Although the exact cause of migraine is unknown, it is suspected to be genetic. Researchers are still examining the complex chain of events in the brain and body of a migraine sufferer immediately before and during a migraine attack. We do know that migraine is a neurobiochemical medical disorder that makes its victims prone to painful attacks. These attacks can be set off in response to migraine triggers.

Q: What are the triggers of migraine?
A: Although the potential triggers of migraine are almost too many to list, types of common triggers include dietary (chocolate, mature cheese, red wine), hormonal (puberty, menstruation), environmental (glare, weather patterns), stress-related (come-down from stress), change-related (changes in sleep patterns or meal times).

Triggers can be external (caused by influences from the outside, such as bright sunlight or foods which are consumed) or internal (caused by influences from within, such as fluctuations in female hormones). Triggers are very individual – what acts as a migraine trigger for one person will not act as a trigger for all. It is important that a person with migraine isolate his or her own triggers or combinations of triggers and avoid them if possible.

Q: I've never been able to isolate particular triggers. Is it okay for me to eat and do whatever I want?
A: Migraine triggers rarely work alone. It is usually in combination that triggers lead to a migraine attack. As well, the body's reaction to triggers can be delayed by 48 hours or more. This makes positive identification of triggers difficult. In general terms, migraine sufferers will create a relatively migraine-friendly environment for themselves by adopting regular eating and sleeping schedules, by participating in regular exercise, by avoiding the more sure-fire migraine foods (such as red wine, mature cheese, chocolate and preservative-rich foods) and by gaining the upper hand on undue stress. These measures will also improve the person's overall health and happiness.

Q: What is the difference between tension headache and migraine?
A: So-called tension headache is usually mild, infrequent and easily remedied through rest or simple non-prescription pain relievers (although chronic tension-type headaches can be debilitating and require medical attention). Migraine tends be more frequent and severe and has more symptoms than common tension-type headache.

'Migraine' is not another word for a bad headache. The

symptoms of migraine are diverse and may include nausea, vomiting, visual disturbances and profound sensitivity to light and sound, in addition to the typical head pain that most people associate with migraine. Anyone with recurring or severe head pain of any sort should see a doctor for diagnosis. The proper diagnosis is needed to ensure that appropriate treatment is given.

Q: This may sound crazy, but before my bad headaches start, I see a checkerboard pattern before my eyes. Once I had a blind spot for about twenty minutes before an attack started. Could this be part of migraine?

A: About 20 per cent of migraine sufferers will, from time to time, experience a neurological warning sign before the onset of their migraine attack. This is called 'migraine with aura'. Commonly the sufferer experiences aura in the form of visual disturbances, but numbness and tingling in an arm or hand or around the mouth, and other symptoms, are possible. It is best to speak to your doctor about your symptoms.

Q: I went to see my doctor about my headaches. I had a CAT scan and it came back normal. Does this mean I'm imagining my migraines?

A: Absolutely not. Migraine is a neurobiochemical disorder of the brain. Migraine occurs right within the blood vessels and nerves of the brain, and can't be seen on an X-ray, scan or routine blood test. Your doctor ordered a scan to rule out the presence of what doctors call 'lesions'. The scan wasn't done to find migraine. So a negative result on your scan reinforces the fact that you may well be suffering from migraine. Ask your doctor for absolute clarification of the diagnosis.

Q: Is migraine hereditary?

A: Migraine tends to run in families. More than half of migraine sufferers can identify a close blood relative who also suffers from migraine (frequently it is their mother). Recent findings by geneticists are outlined in Chapter 1.

Q: Is it possible to have a migraine almost all the time for months, even years?

A: It is possible to have an unremitting headache for long periods. In almost 90 per cent of cases of chronic daily headache, overuse of pain relievers is involved. If pain medication is taken on four or more days per week for an extended period, a condition called 'medication-induced headache' results. These headaches tend to be duller or less intense than migraine headaches, but can drain the joy out of living. Most sufferers of medication-induced headache are unaware of the negative effect that the regular use of pain medication is having on their system; many will deny that their medication intake is a problem. Other related symptoms can include vague dizziness, inability to concentrate, a headache which is present upon waking in the morning, forgetfulness, irritability, sleep disturbances and anxiety or depression. The headache can be brought on by even the slightest intellectual effort.

There is help available, and the cycle of analgesic overuse can be broken. See Chapter 3 for more information.

Q: What is the best medication to take for migraine?

A: No single medication is completely effective, absolutely free of potential side effects and safe for all to take. Taking medication is also not the first step in good migraine management. To gain control over migraine, begin by obtaining a proper diagnosis of headache type. Then identify and eliminate controllable triggers, while improving your overall physical and emotional health. From there, begin to examine and explore the treatment of migraine, both with and without medication, with the help of a doctor. What works for one person won't necessarily work for the next.

Q: Can migraine be treated with non-prescription medications?

A: Only a few migraine sufferers will obtain relief from the infrequent use of non-prescription medications. Simple pain relievers are often not strong enough to 'break' the attack. If this readily available medication is used too often, it may make the headaches appear more often – see the question about 'migraine almost all the time', above. If you need pain relievers on a regular basis, you should be seeking the help of a doctor, and should not be resorting to self-medication.

Q: Are there any new migraine medications coming down the pipeline?

A: There are at least two other triptan medications being developed for the treatment of attacks in progress – eletriptan and frovatriptan. Other research is being done on the preventive side, with interest in the use of the already-marketed naratriptan for the prevention of menstrual migraine.

Other possibilities to aid in the prevention of migraine include the anti-epileptics gabapentin and topiramate, a calcium-channel blocker currently available in Spain called dotrazine, and two anti-asthma medications – montelukast sodium and zafirlukast – that block leukotriene-inflammatory chemicals suspected to be present during a migraine attack. Finally, the use of botulinum toxin type A injections is being closely investigated.

Q: I'm taking a preventive drug for my migraine along with another pill I can take if an attack breaks through. It seems to be working well, but I don't like the idea of being on the daily preventive medication. Will I have to take the preventive forever?

A: No. Usually the preventive medication is given for some period (frequently about four to six months or more) before a 'holiday' from it. The preventive may not have to be restarted for some time if the migraine symptoms stay in check (occasionally it will never need to be restarted).

Q: Should I be using alternative therapies for my migraine?

A: Over the years, reports and claims have been made concerning a wide variety of alternative therapies for migraine. Although scientific evidence on the effectiveness and ultimate safety of several options is simply not available, you are free to do your own research. Consult your medical doctor before proceeding with alternative therapies.

Q: Does migraine lead to brain tumours?

A: Migraine has no relationship to brain tumours.

Q: Are migraine sufferers more likely than the general population to suffer a stroke?

A: Although very rare types of migraine may be associated with a particular type of stroke, population-based studies indicate that migraine sufferers are not likely to suffer stroke more frequently than non-migraine sufferers.

Q: Is there a cure for migraine?

A: There is no cure for migraine, but many sufferers are able to gain control and reduce their attacks through good migraine management.

Q: Why do I feel better after I vomit during a migraine attack?

A: It is believed that the physical act of vomiting raises the body's serotonin level and may act to relieve an attack in progress.

Q: Why do I sometimes feel depressed or weepy during and right after a migraine attack?

A: Many experts believe that this alteration in mood is part of the neurobiochemical imbalance of migraine.

Q: Before many of my attacks I feel unusually well – full of energy and vigour. When I feel that way, I know I'm feeling 'too good' and am likely to be coming down with a migraine. I also crave chocolate desperately. Am I best to give in to the chocolate craving or to resist it?

A: The question of whether to give in to the craving or not can be answered only through experimentation. You may opt to try it both ways and see what happens. If doing either stops an attack from progressing, you'll have your answer. If neither stops it, it's up to you whether to indulge or not. Many other sufferers experience a similar 'feeling too good' sensation before an attack. This phenomenon is probably related to the shifting serotonin and dopamine levels.

Q: Can migraine sufferers take 'the pill'?

A: There is no simple answer to this question. Women with migraine who wish to take the birth-control pill should discuss it with their doctor. The birth-control pill may aggravate migraine in some cases, or it might have no worsening effects. Some doctors will hesitate to prescribe the pill to migraine sufferers, especially to sufferers of migraine with aura. Women who take the pill should not smoke cigarettes, and this is especially true for those who suffer from migraine.

Q: Can pregnancy make migraine worse?

A: Most migraine sufferers find their migraine stays much the same, or may worsen slightly, during the first three months of pregnancy. However, most migraine sufferers report a reduction in the number of migraine attacks experienced after the first three months. Some expectant mothers will experience a virtual elimination of migraine for the majority of their pregnancy. Unfortunately, this bliss is temporary – the migraine usually returns shortly into the post-partum period.

For a small percentage, migraine will continue or even worsen slightly during the entire pregnancy. The challenges involved in treating migraine in pregnancy include weighing the benefit of using medication against the potential risks the medication may pose to the fetus. Women must consult their doctors for advice regarding any treatments used for migraine in pregnancy (or while breastfeeding).

Q: Can children get migraine?

A: Yes. Estimates are that between 5 and 10 per cent of children will suffer a migraine attack. Often there is a family history of migraine. Before puberty, boys are more likely than girls to get migraine and many children 'outgrow' migraine.

Q: How do I obtain a referral to a clinic or a neurologist who specializes in migraine?

A: Most migraine sufferers start by enlisting the help of their family doctor or general practitioner. Sometimes, but not always, the family doctor will refer you to a consulting neurologist in order to confirm an initial diagnosis, or later on in the treatment if the migraine is resistant to what the doctor has to offer. All neurologists are familiar with migraine; a referral from the doctor is usually needed in order to secure a neurology appointment.

Some migraine sufferers attend migraine clinics. Some clinics specialize in one particular treatment approach (often alternative to mainstream medicine) while others are private, multidisciplinary clinics run by medical doctors.

Q: Should I see a psychiatrist about my headaches?
A: Migraine is not a psychiatric illness, but there is a higher incidence of depression in people with migraine, and a higher incidence of migraine in people with depression. This points to a shared biological root for the two disorders. When they co-exist, each requires diagnosis and custom-tailored treatment. Also, if undue stresses or pressures in life act to trigger attacks in someone who suffers from migraine, counselling may be of help. Behaviour-modification strategies may be helpful to those seeking to control any 'Type A' behaviour that exists.

Q: Will my headaches get worse as I get older?
A: Most people's migraine actually improves during the fifth decade of life. This may be owing to natural changes in brain chemistry associated with ageing. In women, the passing of menopause may have an alleviating effect.

Q: What eyeglasses are best to filter out light?
A: A study done with children in Britain reported that rose-tinted glasses reduce headaches triggered by indoor fluorscent lighting. Individuals have reported relief from wearing amber-coloured glasses to cut down on the glare of approaching car headlights at night. When outdoors during

the day, however, migraine sufferers are wise to sport sunglasses to shade their eyes during and between attacks.

There are many types of sunglasses available. Although prices vary widely, what you are usually paying for is the frame or the designer label on the frame. The effectiveness of the lens is the important part of the glasses, and good inexpensive lenses can be found.

Lenses are often marked with a tag which describes the percentage of both the harmful rays that are blocked and the visible light that is blocked. You should look for percentages based on your activity – for days at the beach on holiday, you'll need high percentages, but for shopping on slightly overcast days you'll need lower percentages. During an attack, you'll probably need a very dark pair if you must venture out into bright sunlight. Often it is a matter of personal preference and comfort. Consult an optometrist, ophthalmologist or optician if in doubt.

Q: Is there a preferred place in the world where a migraine sufferer should live to avoid attacks?

A: Headache is prevalent around the world with more than 70 per cent of women in Europe affected by headache at age 40. Some studies have shown migraine to be more prevalent at higher altitudes. Others believe migraine is more prevalent around large bodies of water, owing to more dramatic weather fluctuations. But, practically speaking, since weather patterns vary everywhere on the planet, and weather is not by any means the only factor involved in migraine, moving away is more likely to disrupt your life and cause financial strain than it is to reduce migraine attacks significantly.

These topics are covered in more complete detail in earlier chapters of this book.

Table of Drug Names

Generic name	Some common brand names
Paracetamol*	Atasol, Tempra, Tylenol
Acetylsalicylic acid	Aspergum, Aspirin
Amitriptyline	Elavil
Atenolol	Tenormin
Botulinum toxin type A	Botox
Butorphanol tartrate	Stadol NS
Chlorpromazine	Largactil, Thorazine
Citalopram	Cipramil
Clonidine	Catapres
Codeine*	
Cyproheptadine	Periactin
Danazol	Cyclomen, Danocrine
Diclofenac sodium	Cataflam, Voltaren
Dihydroergotamine mesylate (DHE)	Dihydroergotamine, D.H.E.45
Diltiazem	Cardizem, Dilacor-XR
Domperidone maleate	Motilium
Doxepin	Sinequan, Triadapin
Ergotamine tartrate*	Ergomar, Ergostat
Flunarizine	Sibelium
Fluoxetine	Prozac
Flurbiprofen	Ansaid, Froben
Fluvoxamine	Luvox
Gabapentin	Neurontin
Ibuprofen	Advil, Motrin, Nuprin
Indomethacin	Indocid, Indocin
Isometheptene mucate	Midrid
Ketoprofen	Orudis, Oruvail, Rhodis
Ketorolac	Toradol
Mefenamic acid	Ponstan, Ponstel
Methadone hydrochloride	Methadose
Methysergide maleate	Sansert
Metoclopramide	Clopra, Maxeran, Reglan
Metoprolol	Betaloc, Lopressor, Toprol-XL
Montelukast sodium	Singulair
Morphine sulfate	MS Contin, MS-1R, M.O.S.-Sulfate

Nadolol	Corgard
Nafarelin acetate	Synarel
Naproxen	Naprosyn, Naxen
Naproxen sodium	Anaprox, Synflex, Aleve
Naratriptan	Amerge
Nortriptyline	Aventyl, Pamelor
Oxycodone hydrochloride*	Oxycontin
Paroxetine	Paxil
Pentazocine	Talwin
Phenelzine sulfate	Nardil
Pizotifen	Sandomigran, Sandomigran DS
Prochlorperazine	Compazine, Stemetil
Propranolol	Inderal
Raloxifene	Evista
Rizatriptan	Maxalt
Sertraline	Zoloft
Sumatriptan	Imitrex
Timolol maleate	Blocadren
Topiramate	Topamax
Verapamil	Calan, Isoptin, Verelan
Zafirlukast	Accedate, Accolate
Zolmitriptan	Zomig

Paracetamol, aspirin, codeine and caffeine are present, singularly or in combination, in many over-the-counter and prescription painkillers. Check package labels and inserts, or ask your chemist, to find out exactly what these combination products contain.

Further Resources

World Headache Alliance

More than 40 headache organizations from over 30 nations worldwide have recently come together to form the unprecedented global co-operative World Headache Alliance (WHA).

The Alliance aims to improve the lives of people with headache throughout the world by sharing information among existing headache organizations and by fostering the development of new headache organizations in areas where none currently exists. Together, these organizations seek to increase the awareness and understanding of headache as a public health concern with profound social and economic impact.

WHA member organizations are working side by side with the best headache researchers, scientists and clinicians today. WHA is working closely with the professionally based International Headache Society (IHS) (www.i-h-s.org) towards jointly fostering relationships with the World Health

Organization in Geneva, Switzerland, in order to ensure that headache disorders receive full attention worldwide.

For websites and up-to-the-minute information, check out the World Headache Alliance's website at www.ihaveaheadache.com.

Patient-based migraine organizations

Migraine Action Association
Unit 6, Oakley Hay Lodge Business Park
Great Folds Road
Great Oakley, Northants
NN18 9AS
Tel (01536) 461333
Fax (01536) 461444
info@migraine.org.uk
www.migraine.org.uk

The Migraine Trust
45 Great Ormond Street
London
WCIN 3H2
Tel (0207) 831 4818
Fax (0207) 831 5174
info@migrainetrust.org
www.migrainetrust.org

Glossary

Analgesic: Pain-relieving medication.

Antiemetic: Medication used to relieve nausea and/or prevent vomiting.

Aura: The term used for neurological events which may occur before a migraine attack in approximately 20 per cent of migraine sufferers from time to time. Some people equate aura with a warning sign.

Beta-adrenergic blockers: A specific class of medication which sometimes helps reduce the frequency of migraine attacks if taken on a daily basis. The precise reason why beta blockers are effective for some people is unknown, but they are believed to block underlying chemical disruptions within the brain.

Biofeedback: Short for 'biological feedback', biofeedback is a technique for trying to control the body's biological responses, learned by using feedback from electronic devices.

Brain stem: The part of the brain that connects the spinal cord to the two sides of the brain.

Calcium-channel blockers:
A type of medication intended to reduce the frequency and/or severity of migraine attacks when taken daily. Calcium-channel blockers help prevent excess calcium ions from crossing into muscle cells in the arteries, rendering them less likely to spasm and cause a migraine attack. They do not rob the body of necessary calcium.

CAT scan: The computerized axial tomography, or CAT, scan offers a painless look into the brain with the help of computer technology. CAT scans are often enhanced by the injection of a contrast dye into the patient. In migraine, the results of a CAT scan will usually be negative. Also called 'CT scan'.

Cephalalgia (or Cephalgia):
Head pain.

Clinician: A medical doctor who deals directly with patients, rather than with research, etc.

Cluster headache: Attacks of severe, one-sided pain around the eye, above the eye, or in the region of the temple which last from 15 minutes to three hours characterize cluster headache. These painful attacks occur from once every other day up to eight times per day. Cluster headache derives its name from the pattern of attacks, which occur in clusters lasting for weeks or months, separated by periods of remission which can last months or years. 'Chronic cluster headache' (where there is no remission) occurs in about 10 per cent of cluster sufferers.

Ergotamine: A medication used to constrict blood vessels.

Hemiplegia: A paralysis of one side of the body (can be temporary or permanent – most often temporary if migraine-related).

Hypoglycaemia: Low blood sugar.

Medication-induced headache: A type of headache disorder caused by withdrawal from the regular overuse of pain-relieving or ergot-containing preparations or caffeine. Also called 'rebound headache'.

Migraine with aura: An aura is a neurological disturbance commonly characterized by unusual phenomena ranging from seeing flashing lights and blank spots in the field of vision to feeling numbness and tingling in the fingers or around the mouth. *See also* **Aura**.

Migraine without aura: A recurring headache disorder which causes attacks lasting from 4 to 72 hours. The typical throbbing head pain of a migraine attack is almost always accompanied by other symptoms such as nausea, vomiting and heightened sensitivity to light and sound, among others.

Migraineur: A person who suffers from migraine.

MRI: A sophisticated form of scan called 'magnetic resonance imaging' that has recently become available in many larger hospitals. The MRI offers more detail than a CAT scan, but is more expensive and less readily available. In migraine, the MRI results will probably be negative.

Neuralgia: Pain caused by inflammation of a nerve.

Neurogenic: Originating in the nervous system.

Neurotransmitter: Naturally occurring chemicals that are released at nerve endings to pass messages from one nerve ending to the next.

Oedema: Swelling.

Oestrogen: A female sex hormone.

PET: Positron emission tomography, which uses a camera to measure metabolic, functional and biochemical activity in brain tissue after the injection of a small amount of radioactive material.

Phonophobia: Heightened sensitivity to sound.

Photophobia: Heightened sensitivity to light.

Prophylactic medication: Also known as 'preventive' medication, this class of drug is taken on a daily basis to help correct the chemical imbalances in the brain that underpin migraine.

Serotonin: A neurotransmitter or naturally occurring chemical messenger believed to play an important role in migraine.

Tension-type headache: Tension-type headache causes recurrent episodes of headache lasting from minutes to days. The head pain is often described as 'band-like' or 'pressing' and can make the sufferer feel as if he or she is wearing a hat that is much too tight. The pain is mild or moderate, and is felt on both sides of the head. The pain does not worsen with physical movement, and although sufferers may be sensitive to light or sound, they are not nauseated.

Triggers: Internal and external factors that can act to set a migraine in motion. Triggers are individual, and what affects one person will not necessarily affect another. Common categories of triggers include dietary triggers; hormonal factors; changes in usual routines, meal times and sleep times; stress or the come-down period from stress; and environmental factors such as the weather.

Triptans: A group of prescription medications that affect the behaviour of the nerve chemical serotonin. Triptans are used to treat migraine attacks in progress.

Tyramine: A chemical found in mature cheese and other foods that is capable of causing a dilation (widening) of blood vessels, resulting in migraine in susceptible people.

Vascular: Pertaining to the blood vessels.

Vasoconstriction: A narrowing of the blood vessels.

Vasodilation: A widening of the blood vessels.

Acknowledgements
with Admiration and Thanks

City of London Migraine Clinic
Dr E. Anne MacGregor MB BS MFFP
Director of Clinical Research

Migraine Association of Canada's
Medical Advisory Committee

Marek J. Gawel MA MB BCh FRCPUK FRCPC
Director, Headache Research Institute, Sunnybrook and
*   Women's College Health Sciences Centre, Toronto, ON*
Secretary and Ex-President, Canadian Headache Society

Elie Cass BA MD *Family Physician, Toronto, ON*

R. Allan Purdy MD FRCPC
Head, Division of Neurology, Department of Medicine,
*   Dalhousie University, Halifax, NS*
Chief of Neurology Service, Queen Elizabeth Health
*   Sciences Centre, Halifax, NS*

President, Canadian Headache Society

R. Gordon Robinson BSc MD FRCPC
Clinical Associate Professor, Division of Neurology,
  University of British Columbia
Medical Manager, Neurology, Vancouver Hospital and
  Health Sciences Centre, Vancouver, BC

Ashfaq Shuaib MD FRCPC
Professor of Medicine, Director of Neurology, University
  of Alberta, Edmonton, AB

Irene Worthington BSc Phm
Coordinator, Metro Toronto Hospitals Drug Information
  Service, Sunnybrook and Women's College Health
  Sciences Centre, Toronto, ON

American Council for Headache Education (ACHE)
Fred D. Sheftell MD (National President)
Director and Founder, New England Centre for Headache,
  Stamford, CT
Clinical Assistant Professor, New York Medical College,
  Valhalla, NY

Contributors

Chapter 9, 'The Triptans', was written by Dr Marek J.
  Gawel (see above).

Chapter 5, 'Migraine in Infants and Children,' includes
  contributions from the following:

Daune L. MacGregor MD
Professor of Paediatrics (Neurology), University of
  Toronto
Staff Neurologist, Hospital for Sick Children, Toronto, ON

J.M. Dooley MB FRCPC
Associate Professor of Pediatrics, Dalhousie University,
* Halifax, NS*
Chief, Division of Neurology, IWK Health Centre,
* Halifax, NS*

Wendy Gage MSW
Department of Neurology, Hospital for Sick Children,
* Toronto, ON*

Index